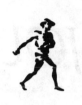

JOURNEY

OF A DIABETIC

◆ ◆ ◆

by Lawrence M. Pray

with Richard Evans III, M.D.

SIMON AND SCHUSTER

NEW YORK

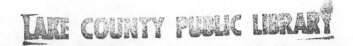

16668535

Library of Congress Cataloging in Publication Data
Pray, Lawrence M.
Journey of a diabetic.
1. Diabetics—United States—Biography.   2. Pray,
Lawrence M.   I. Evans, Richard, date-   II. Title.
RC660.P74   1983   362.1'96462'0924 [B]   82-19276
ISBN 0-671-45396-3

To my family

✦ CONTENTS ✦

POSTSCRIPTS

✦ ACKNOWLEDGMENTS ✦

I scarcely know where to begin in offering my thanks to those who helped make this journey possible. I wish I could meet again with the doctors, kids, relatives, teachers, camps, ministers, schools, and coaches whose friendship, comments, teachings, and impressions have stayed with me throughout the years. Some of you know how important you have been, and others may not realize the impact you made with a simple comment until you find yourself in the book. In either case, I hope I have captured correctly the spirit of your teaching and offer my heartfelt thanks.

Thanks go to my brothers and parents for their support and willingness to tell a straight story. Diabetes is a family affair, and without their help the book couldn't have been written.

A special thanks goes to Lynn Caine. When this book was an idea that "just had to happen," she gave the guidance and support that introduced me to the world of publishing. I've often called her the book's godmother, and am deeply grateful for her help.

The partnership of Dick Evans in the entire project has been especially invaluable. The many evenings we spent together added a depth and objectivity that I couldn't have had alone, and I value the relationship we've developed a great deal.

Dr. Alan Jacobson of the Joslin Clinic and Dr. Dan Wood of Bath were both very helpful in their review of the manuscript, and their suggestions have been applied.

I'd also like to thank Peter Skolnik, who has been both agent and guide par excellence throughout this entire project. He saw that the book "could happen" and has been of immense help. I am also appreciative of the experience and patience of my editor, Peter Schwed, whose fine criticism kept the book on course.

My thanks to the Hyde School in its pioneering days for its support and its quest for excellence and commitment in education. Finally, my deepest appreciation goes to my wife and four kids, to whom I'm pleased to report that the book really is finally finished.

Bath, Maine
September 1982

• INTRODUCTION •

The fact that I remember few experiences before turning diabetic has always struck me as odd. Nearly seven years were tucked away somewhere, but waking up in the Rumford hospital felt like the real beginning. It led me to a reluctant conclusion. While I might have liked to say that diabetes is just another part of my life, the fact is that it touched me and my family far more than any of us realized.

Over the next twenty-two years, coming to terms with diabetes became an almost epic struggle. It was something I wanted to control but couldn't, wanted to tuck away into a private corner and quietly forget. But every time I tried, it snapped right back. Diabetes controlled me more than I controlled diabetes. When I finally mentioned my difficulties to my doctor, he said, "We call that accepting the disease." He was right. But how do you accept?

Diabetes presented a dilemma that couldn't be resolved through logical, conventional wisdom. On the one hand, it needed to be carefully monitored and controlled. Several shots a day, regular urine testings, steady exercise, eating a precise number of calories at each and every meal, special foot-care rules, and maintaining a consistent daily routine all needed to be kept in mind. At the same time, we were told that through control we could lead perfectly normal lives. It felt like a trap. Compliance with the exacting rules sparked an almost instinctive rebellion; yet poor control led to illness. I was caught between a compliance I couldn't buy and a denial that wouldn't work. Like many diabetics, I ended up with an excellent understanding of how things "should be" and a poor understanding of how to get there.

In some ways it was both a cultural and a personal problem. Disease is quite naturally seen as an enemy. When polio was virtually eliminated, we rejoiced. The same was true with smallpox. But what happens when the disease is incurable, and you must accept what you have been taught to conquer? It's no wonder growing up with diabetes is an exercise in contradictions.

Eventually, however, there came a kind of breakthrough once I saw that juvenile diabetes wasn't the enemy I'd feared. When I fully realized that it needn't be separated from the rest of my life, and that accepting diabetes wasn't giving in to a weakness, it changed from an enemy and became a teacher.

Learning one of the greatest lessons of my life was often a lonely experience. The acceptance process that every diabetic inevitably faces was generally ignored. It was as though diabetics were supposed to automatically possess the willing attitude, great wisdom, and sense of restraint that would make acceptance easy. Admirable as those qualities were, they sure didn't reflect the way I grew up. How could anybody be that perfect and still maintain a sense of his individuality? When I ran into accounts written by young or old diabetics saying their diabetes didn't interfere with their lives in the least, their stories struck me as suspect. I had once said the same kind of thing, but now realize it was true only on the surface.

How diabetics "really" grew up and came to terms with their disease remained a mystery. Available books offered solutions that spoke to my disease but never to my life. And although acceptance was the one challenge that linked all diabetics together, nobody talked about just how one actually learns to accept. Realizing how meaningful acceptance eventually was for me, and thinking I might have benefited if I'd read a true story, I decided to offer my experience in the hope that diabetics and their families could take increased faith in their journey with disease.

I was talking one evening about my plans for the book with Richard Evans, who had stopped by the school for dinner. As a friend and as a psychiatrist, he became intrigued with the idea, and by the end of the evening we had decided to join forces. He brought an objectivity I clearly didn't have, as well as a professional and personal curiosity. He began with the hunch that a young diabetic's struggle with acceptance is similar to problems all young people face as they mature. As we progressed, we found that diabetes both accelerates and clarifies the challenges inherent in growing up.

Over the next year I recounted the stories that were most vivid in my memory. He listened, asked questions, and explored with me the stages of growth and acceptance. We both realized we needed to find a balance between those experiences which were important to me as a person and those which related only to diabetes. Only by weaving together my life and my diabetes could the story of acceptance be told. After all, diabetes influenced my growth just as my growth influenced diabetes, and acceptance was a matter of reconciling the two.

We recognized that juvenile diabetes has as profound an influence on the family of a diabetic as it does on the diabetic himself. My wife, Connie, helped explore diabetes in our marriage, and at a Christmas gathering I asked my parents and three younger brothers for help. They wanted to do their part, and we spent a family evening sharing our experiences with diabetes for the first time in twenty-five years.

I should add that this book is a story of personal recollections and understandings. I have not interviewed thousands of diabetics as a researcher might. The diabetics I've met over the years probably aren't much different from those in your own community. Coming to an acceptance means drawing on the human resources that are as available to you as they were to me. While my experiences are quite naturally different from yours, the journey toward acceptance is something we share. More than we may realize, it makes us who we are as people.

For me, diabetes is no longer the enemy. It has become a teacher that helps guide me in my growth. Perhaps because acceptance was anything but a superficial process, it has been a rewarding journey. My great-grandfather once said that the main idea in life is to keep your head in the clouds and your feet on the ground. I never had too much difficulty with the cloud part, but the second half was tough. What would I be like if I weren't diabetic? I don't know. But I'm thankful to have my feet on the ground.

In the middle of the journey of our life, I came to myself within a dark wood where the straight way was lost.

—Dante

1 • SEPARATION

It began with a trip to Maine in the summer of 1954. I'd just finished the second grade, had traveled from California to New Jersey to meet my grandparents, and was slated to be their sole guest on the drive to Maine. I was their firstborn grandchild, saw them only rarely, and was leaving my parents for the first time. It was to be an unforgettable trip that marked the beginning of a distinct and profound separation.

My grandfather drove a blue 1953 Chrysler. He called it a lemon, but treated it with careful and painstaking pride. Whereas our family cars were always a mess, he kept the blue Chrysler neat as a pin. I sat in the back seat as we pulled out of the driveway and drove through the streets of Morristown. Once on the highway, we both watched the speedometer's gold needle move up to 60 and then hold steady.

"We're going a mile a minute," he said as he glanced back at me.

"A mile a minute?" I said. It was hard to believe that anything could move that fast. I tried to figure it out for myself, and sure enough, sixty miles an hour meant a mile a minute. It was the kind of event that happened only in the company of grandparents. Maybe I'd traveled that fast before, but it didn't seem like it. I settled back in my seat wondering how the world could pass by so fast.

We pulled into Rye, New Hampshire, late that afternoon, and my Uncle Henry and Aunt Emily were waiting for us. He had coached track at Exeter for many years, and was greatly admired by my mother. The fact that he was a coach scared me a little, because I didn't consider myself much of an athlete and worried that he might ask me how strong I was. Fortunately, he didn't ask.

We'd talked about lobster on the way up, and once we had unpacked and cleaned up we all went out to a summer restaurant on the shore. The hostess showed us onto an outdoor porch, and we chose a long wooden table that faced the sea. There was no need to carefully read the menu, as we all knew exactly what we wanted. My grandfather proudly placed the order, and everyone sat back to relax.

The adults talked about times past, about people I didn't know, about the Academy, my grandfather's box factory, and how much they loved Maine. Although I had been sitting all day, I was remarkably tired and hungry, and it seemed as though the lobsters would never arrive. As we waited and they kept talking, I reached cautiously for the celery, olives, and carrots on a small relish tray. From my seat, I could look out over the ocean behind my grandparents.

It seemed so quiet. Stories I had read about the ocean always pictured it raging, with waves as high as houses and winds that never stopped. But it wasn't that way at all. Although it seemed that a big ocean should have a dramatic edge, it didn't. It was calm and almost flat. The water barely moved, and I could scarcely hear the lapping of the waves.

When we were finally brought the plates of steaming red lobsters, we all leaned back, marveled at the sight, and teased each other as we put on the huge red-and-white bibs. I quickly became the center of attention. How was a seven-year-old boy going to eat a lobster that was half as big as he was? Had I ever seen a lobster before? Was it going to move? Did I know it had actually been boiled alive?

I could hardly wait to begin eating. The adults showed me how to crack the claws and told me to begin. By the time the others were halfway through their lobsters, I had already finished mine and stacked the remains on a separate plate. To everyone's amazement, including my own, I even ate the green tomalley after making sure it really was edible. It struck me that no matter how much I ate or drank, I couldn't fill myself. The food just didn't seem to stick. So as the others finished their meal, I politely asked if I couldn't have another lobster.

"Another lobster?" they asked.

"Yes," I said.

"Do you mean a seven-year-old boy is going to eat not one but two New Hampshire lobsters?" they said. No one had ever heard of such a thing. They laughed, and I knew instantly it had been the wrong thing to ask. Everyone was pleased with my appetite, but one lobster would have to be enough. I agreed, and the adults returned to their conversation. They must have thought I was joking, I thought, but I wasn't. I was still hungry, had told them, but they hadn't heard me. It was as though we were in two different worlds and for some reason I couldn't get through. I reached for a few more crackers, drank another glass of water, and waited for the meal to end.

After dinner we returned to Uncle Henry's house. I must have looked tired by then, because although it was still light out they thought I should turn in. My aunt showed me up to an attic room whose window overlooked the street. It was a New England window, with small panes of glass divided by white crosspieces. I said good night, lay down on the cot, and tried to go to sleep as thoughts went through my mind of the dinner and the thin hunger that wouldn't go away.

After a while I stood up, walked over to the window, and looked down on the people coming and going in the cool of the summer evening. They were laughing and talking, walking down the other side of the street. As I stood there, a feeling came over me that something was wrong. I couldn't pin it down, and scarcely had words for it, but I deeply sensed that something I couldn't understand was wrong. I kept watching the people pass along the sidewalk and wondered what it would be like to share their ease. If I were on that sidewalk I knew I wouldn't belong. Without understanding why, I was different. There was a great distance between us as I sensed that I would never be like them, that I'd never be the same. The difference, whatever it was, carried with it a tinge of fear, a certain sadness, but also a distinction I would never trade.

I do not remember returning to the cot. Nor do I remember the next morning when we loaded up the blue Chrysler and headed on to Maine. But the memory of that window has stayed with me as a strength and as an Achilles' heel throughout my life. It is my first memory as a diabetic.

2 ◆ KEEPING UP

There used to be a giant yellow sardine man that greeted everyone passing from New Hampshire into Maine. As soon as we saw him standing there, we let out a cheer. We had arrived at last, and suddenly the trees looked greener, wilder, and the forests deeper.

My grandparents' cottage was on the shore of Lake Webb, near Rumford. Each summer they vacationed there, leaving the box factory and New Jersey far behind. We called the cottage Pine Hill. It was set amid towering red pines and had a small stone deck that overlooked the lake and its surrounding mountains. Each evening the family would gather on the deck to watch the sun settle into a gap between the blue mountains and to await the first stars. The smell of pine was sharp, and everything in and around the cabin had its own special aura. The cottage itself was filled with secret compartments; it had a stone hearth with faces in it, pine knots that looked to a small boy like animal eyes in the night, and plenty of grown-up-looking life jackets and fishing gear. It all had a specialness that had to be appreciated and well maintained. That's where the problems began.

I couldn't stop having to go to the bathroom. It seemed that every time I turned around I had to relieve myself. I'd go once, urge out every last possible drop, and then say to myself, "There, that should be enough." But it wasn't. An hour later I'd have to go again.

While I knew something was out of the ordinary, I was scared to tell my grandparents. It wasn't that I didn't trust them, because I did.

But they represented the world the way it should be, and I didn't want them to know something unusual was going on. That was easier said than done, because while the cabin had a toilet, it made a lot of noise. If I flushed every time I used it, not only would I be using up all the water, but they'd hear and ask why I was using the bathroom so much. If I didn't flush, even though the urine was almost as pale as water, they still might find out.

Fortunately, there was a woodpile behind the cabin. My best option was to sneak out back and make it a second bathroom. I'd quietly slip out of the house, head for the woodpile without attracting attention, find an ancient pile of logs that no one would ever use, and relieve myself. No one ever saw me; no one ever found out when ten or fifteen times a day I left the cabin and quietly headed for the woodpile. It felt as if I were working double time just to keep afloat.

I was also losing weight—which didn't make sense because I was constantly eating. Here again I was afraid to tell my grandparents just how hungry I was. When I'd tried in New Hampshire no one had seemed to hear me, and I didn't want to be a pest. My grandmother, who generally had a maid cook the meals in New Jersey, was not a fabulous cook, and the meals she served were polite but petite. One night I finished my plate and asked for a second portion of peas. She was thrilled I liked them and commented on my healthy appetite. I ate them with a vengeance, despite the fact that I really didn't like cold peas at all. No matter how much I ate, I'd end up starving.

And thirsty. That was the toughest problem of all. Because we couldn't drink the lake water and didn't have a well, we had to go to a spring five or six miles from the cottage to collect water in huge green-tinged glass bottles. These were turned upside down in a metal frame in the kitchen, and when we wanted a drink we would fill a glass by pressing a small button. The water was excellent, but it was scarce. Two bottles had to last us three days, and I was constantly thirsty.

Somehow I had to make it between collection days without taking more than my fair share of water. I'd take a glass and, just as I had in the bathroom, tell myself it should be enough. But it never was, and with each glass the water level dropped. Even small sips couldn't forestall the inevitable thirst.

Milk and juice were the alternatives, but with them I had the same problem. How much milk could I take without calling attention to myself? Then I thought of a plan. One night I said I didn't like warm milk, and asked if I couldn't add some ice cubes. My grandmother was surprised, but agreed. My plan had worked. The ice cubes gave me water, stretched the milk, and moved us all that much closer to a new bottle of water.

My grandparents loved me deeply, and I'm sure that had I told them something was wrong they would have been the first people on earth to help me out. But I wouldn't have known what to say, because I scarcely knew myself what was going on. The thought that I might be sick never crossed my mind. When my mother arrived at Pine Hill I didn't say anything to her either. I was being overwhelmed by something I still had no words for. The worse it became the more I held on to appearances. I didn't want to cause problems, to empty the water I knew was scarce, to use the bathroom more than I should, to complain. Day after day I fought to keep up.

Noticing my weight loss, my grandparents suspected I was home-sick. They presumed that my mother's presence would get things back to normal. My mother must have assumed the same thing, because it was several days before she called a local doctor. He took some blood and urine specimens and said he'd call back with the results.

"I was at the beach swimming," my mother said, recalling the afternoon the doctor called back. "Somebody called and said the doctor was on the phone and had the results of the tests. I went to the cottage, still in a wet bathing suit, and talked to him on the phone. Before he told me, he said, 'Do you have any clue, Mrs. Pray, about what is the matter with your son? What do you think it might be?' That was exactly the way he started the conversation.

" 'Well,' I said, 'I think it's a reaction he probably has from a polio shot he had in California.' And there was this really mysterious, long silence. I think he knew from the very moment he told me that our lives would be different. And he wanted to keep putting it off just one more minute. Then he finally said, 'No, he has diabetes.' "

The word set off a flurry of panic in everyone. My grandparents felt that perhaps if they'd called the doctor sooner, or if perhaps they'd been more attentive during the trip to Maine, the diagnosis could have been changed or prevented. And there was fear. My grandmother's niece, who had the queer nickname of Tweet, had died of diabetes in the early 1900s.

My grandparents worried about my mother; my father was three thousand miles away, in a remote geology field camp in the Zuni Mountains; and everyone worried about me. In the midst of the commotion, my mother forged ahead as best as she could.

"The only person who could be strong," said my mother, "was me. There was no way of reaching your dad. And my mother and father were not the kind of parents to break down in front of. I certainly couldn't let my feelings go with you. I just didn't think that was the thing to do. So my role immediately became: 'Now, look, everybody, there is absolutely nothing to this. We are able to handle it, whatever "it" is.' "

She gathered together a few things for me and we set out for the hospital in Rumford. For the first time I knew I was more than different. I was very sick. I had lost my energy, and the whole matter seemed out of my hands. My mother dressed me in a bright red shirt that seemed too big. For some reason it wasn't a shirt I would have chosen to wear, and to this day I still shy away from bright red shirts. They carried me to the blue Chrysler and laid me down on the back seat. We pulled up the forest lane and onto the road to Rumford. My mother drove as I dozed and slept, trying to keep out the fear. I felt as though I were being transported to another world.

3 · THE BEGINNING

The hospital room was pale yellow, its windows wide and high. The yellow curtains ran from the heat register to the ceiling. There were four or five beds in the room, some filled, some empty, and in the mornings the whole room was flooded with warm sunlight. I was not afraid of that room. When I awoke in it, I felt as if I had returned.

There was no long recovery. I simply woke up and everything seemed full, open, and remarkably alive. It was as though senses I had lost or had firmly held in check had returned full force. Whatever was wrong had left me; I felt like myself again.

On the far side of the room was a farm boy named Caroll. In California no boy would ever be named Caroll, but my mother told me on one of her visits that Caroll was indeed a man's name and was common in Maine. His right arm was in a cast. He had been baling hay when he fell and caught it in the baler. He seemed very brave about it. He was about my age, and when he talked about the accident I had visions of a giant machine pulling him into its gears and noise, of his family frantically trying to stop the machine before it took all of him. The cast went from his wrist clear to his shoulder.

"What's wrong with *you*?" he asked.

"I'm diabetic," I said, "but I feel fine."

"How long will you be here?"

"Not long. How about you?"

"I'm supposed to be home in a few days, but the cast has to be on for six weeks."

24

And then we began the long discussions. The question was whether it was better to have your arm broken in a baler or be a diabetic who feels fine but who will be diabetic much longer than six weeks. I think we both decided it was better to be a diabetic, but suspect we both wanted to trade.

From time to time our families would visit. His family always came in shy groups. They must have felt awful about his getting his arm caught in the baler. They'd stay for a short while, tell him what was happening at home, wish him well, and then leave. And my mother would come. She would sit beside my bed working on a quilt. Its sections were hand-sewn, each made of colorful patches cut into small triangles that reminded me of kaleidoscope patterns. We didn't talk much, but there was a closeness between us as I sat in bed gathering my strength and she sat in the sun sewing and keeping me quiet company.

I still had no idea what the word "diabetic" meant. All I knew was that I had awakened from a frightening condition. I no longer needed to urinate every other moment, my thirst had returned to normal, and food strengthened me. My doctor, Dr. Holland, was the epitome of a Maine country doctor. He was at least in his eighties (or so he seemed to me), with white hair, a black medical bag, and a voice of gentle authority. I liked him. Whatever he had done had worked, and he could be trusted.

It's odd that I don't remember the first shots or any fear of being diabetic. He told me I needed to take care of myself, and I enthusiastically agreed. It struck me as a grand adventure more than anything else. The thought that maybe I didn't want to be diabetic hadn't entered my mind. The shots, the urine tests, and my friend Dr. Holland were all allies on the side of life.

I took 6 units of NPH U-40, one of the most frequently used forms of insulin. The shot, which replaced the insulin my body was supposed to produce, was to be taken each morning. He told me too much or too little insulin, too much or too little food, would throw my diabetes off balance and I'd end up feeling just as I had before entering the hospital. He taught me to check the sugar in my urine as a way to monitor my control. I agreed to follow his every direction, though I had no idea how insulin, diet, urine tests, and exercise all connected. He gave me and my mother charts that specified what to eat, when to eat it, and how much to eat at every meal. He told us to keep careful records, and to come back and see him at the end of the week. We left the hospital, and launched into diabetes with a crusadelike spirit.

Life took on new routines, and the cover-ups were discarded. I used the bathroom like everyone else, flushed the toilet with confidence, and drank water without a trace of guilt. At three thirty each and every afternoon I ate four saltines and two tablespoons of peanut butter. Anticipating the three-thirty snack was like waiting for the races. We'd all go out on the deck overlooking the lake, carefully measure the peanut butter, and spread it over the crackers. Three thirty became a special time of day for all of us.

My grandfather, the craftsman, cut small blocks of wood shaped like pieces of steak or ground beef. Each represented 30 grams, and we carefully rounded hamburger patties to the size of Grandfather's blocks. We measured the beans, the peas, the pats of butter, and the glasses of milk. We cooked eggs with an exact amount of oil; wondered how we would know what kind of cereal to buy, what we should do if the store apples were too small or too large; and did so without complaining. There was nothing to complain about. I was living life the way it should be, and the precise routines seemed to perfect and strengthen the hope that had returned with Dr. Holland and the Rumford hospital.

At least, that was the way it seemed. Beneath our enthusiasm, however, we fought and lost our first battle with diabetes. My mother and I kept careful track of my urine tests, as they were the best indication of my overall control. Four times a day we recorded them in a small black notebook Dr. Holland would ask for at the end of the week. I had started on 6 units of NPH, and the tests kept showing up negative. The dark blue negative tests meant everything was on track, and we enjoyed watching the pages fill with the encouraging results. Each negative test also meant less insulin was needed. We cut the dosage down to 5, then to 4, then all the way down to 2 units.

Our hopes grew as the units decreased. Two units were hardly worth taking, I told myself. If I followed the doctor's instructions carefully, I was sure that I soon wouldn't need insulin at all. After several days at 2 units, we decided to call Dr. Holland and ask if the shots were really necessary. His answer was direct and discouraging: stay on the insulin.

Perhaps my mother was prepared for it, but I believed he was wrong. I didn't feel bitter or resentful about the shots, the tests, and the diet, and would never complain about the routines that had been so miraculous, but I hoped he was wrong. After all, I had taken perfect care of myself for several weeks, and my body seemed to be saying we had the thing almost licked. Perhaps I could be strong enough and good enough to make it on my own. The next morning I took another 2 units, and I waited for another string of negative tests to take to Dr. Holland.

I couldn't know then that several weeks later the tests would begin to show sugar, and that my dosages of insulin would increase from 2 back to 4, on up to 6, 8, 12, and eventually into hundreds, with two shots a day and two different kinds of insulin. It turns out that the first injections of insulin somehow stimulate the pancreas to produce a last gasp of its own insulin before bowing out, and that's what had happened. I may have spoken to someone about my disappointment, but doubt it. I do remember sitting alone on the deck overlooking the lake and thinking about it. There was really nothing to complain about, but the units slowly moved up, and despite my perfection with shots, saltines, and peanut butter, I moved further and further away from one last injection, one last time.

4 ◆ BREAKING IN

By the time we arrived back in California, the adventure was over, and diabetes became an increasingly standard part of my life. No longer did the family get together for the three-thirty snacks; no longer did I hope the dosage might slip down to zero and disappear. I was diabetic, and there were certain things I had to do.

One of them was to take my own shots. The needle's transition from nurse to my mother was fairly painless, thanks to the diabetic orange. A hospital class for the nervous mothers of new diabetics had taught her the mechanics of injection. An orange, they assured her, had approximately the same texture as the human leg. She could get the hang of giving shots by practicing on the orange, and then use the same technique on me.

It must have worked, because when she gave me my morning shot she did it without a hint of fear or hesitation. However, she quickly determined that I should accept the responsibility of giving myself my own injections and passed the needle on to me.

The needles back then were not the micro-smooth lubricated disposable wonders of today. They were made of tempered steel, were kept sterile in alcohol, and were used over and over again. My father and I would sharpen them on a whetstone. This practice shocked many, but to us it made all the sense in the world. If a whetstone could sharpen a knife blade to within an inch of its life, as my father would say, it could sharpen a needle as well. And it did. I enjoyed sharpening the needles, and kind of liked the alcohol, the Clinitest tablets, and the paraphernalia of diabetes that caught the envy of my younger brothers. But when it came to my actually giving the shots, their envy and my interest disappeared in a hurry.

To help me out, my mother handed me an orange for target practice. It had worked for her, and we both thought it might work for me as well. So I would hold the orange in the palm of my left hand with great confidence. In my right hand was the syringe, loaded with the correct dosage of water. I would hold the syringe about four inches from the orange, squeeze the orange the same way my mother squeezed up the skin on my leg, and then give it a quick jab. It worked every time. The needle passed through the orange skin without the slightest hitch. Neither the orange nor I flinched in the least. Once it was in, I'd push down on the plunger to administer the dose and then pull out the syringe. I'd even wipe the orange with alcohol both before and after the injection to prevent any chance of infection.

I practiced this hundreds and hundreds of times, with unqualified success each time. I suspect there never has been a diabetic who had a problem injecting an orange, nor the parent of a diabetic who flinched from the task. But moving from an orange to my leg changed the name of the game.

To put it mildly, my courage vanished in an instant. I would swab my thigh five or six times with alcohol until it was clean as a whistle. I'd fill the syringe with insulin, double-check the dose, and squeeze up the flesh just as shown in the diabetic book. I'd hold the syringe several inches from my leg and take careful aim. And then I'd freeze. I just couldn't bring myself to do it. I desperately looked over to the kitchen. Breakfast was waiting on the table, the family moved in its own directions on all sides of me, there was a chance I'd be late to school, and there I was stuck on my stool trying to pretend my leg was an orange.

Not knowing what to do, but knowing for sure I wouldn't be bailed out, I yielded to my imagination. I somehow became convinced that the faster the injection, the more it would hurt. This thought had nothing to do with reality. The quick jabs given both in the hospital and by my mother rarely hurt. Just a small prick, hardly

29

even a prick sometimes, and it was over. Logic should have told me that the faster the entry, the less the pain. But such reflections never had a chance. As soon as I held the syringe in my own hand, I became totally convinced that the slower the entry, the less it would hurt. If I could just sneak up on it ever so slowly by pushing it in bit by bit, maybe it would sink beneath the skin and I wouldn't quite know how it got there. And if I squeezed my flesh long enough, maybe it would deaden all the nerve endings and my leg wouldn't even realize a needle was on its way through.

So I held the needle just above my leg and began to slowly, ever so slowly, prepare for the injection. As I squeezed my leg harder and harder, I'd push down just a bit on the point of the needle. If I kept my body, arm, and wrist rigid, and then leaned forward just a touch, the tip would slowly sink in. A little more lean and the needle tip disappeared. A little more and the first eighth of an inch was in the skin. I kept pushing ever so slowly until the entire needle sank beneath the skin. Then I took a deep breath, made sure I didn't jiggle my hand, and pushed down on the plunger, wondering just where the insulin went.

The entire process took at least fifteen minutes. Once I put the syringe back into its metal case and added a little fresh alcohol, I joined everyone at breakfast. My parents must have been glad the ordeal was over, and had probably gone through agony during the entire operation. But they didn't make too big a deal out of it. I'd accomplished what I was supposed to do. They never bailed me out, and I knew that the responsibility rested squarely on my shoulders. Once in a while after a particularly trying morning my mother would suggest in an offhand manner that I should practice some more on an orange. But we knew it was pointless. Pretend as I would, the orange wasn't the same as my leg.

It was my grandfather who came to the rescue. One day a small package arrived for me in the mail. In a rectangular box was a device called an "injector." With it came a short note and an elaborate diagram drawn out on yellow paper. He was a designer of self-opening boxes, and his diagram showed in three dimensions exactly how the syringe fitted into the injector and exactly how it worked.

The injector was actually a kind of spring-powered plunger. The loaded syringe was placed in the injector's chamber and locked into place. The chamber could be pulled back to coil a strong spring. Once the device was cocked, it held the needle just above my skin at exactly the right angle for injection. All I had to do was squeeze my skin a little and push the trigger. The spring would do the rest.

After we figured out how it worked, we pulled out an orange and gave it a try. It worked like a charm. Having nothing to lose, I tried it on myself the next morning. Once everything was in place, I pushed down on the trigger very slowly and waited for it to go off. I kept waiting and waiting for the snap, but when it finally came the needle shot into my leg in an instant. I scarcely felt a thing. Once it was in I pushed down on the plunger with increased confidence, pulled out the whole assembly, and swabbed the entire area with alcohol. It was a lifesaver.

For the next five or six years I used the injector every day. It became an almost automatic process, and I eventually prided myself on being able to do the whole operation in less than a minute. I knew deep down that one day I would have to outgrow it. Easy answers never work, and even then I couldn't help feeling that it was slightly cheating to use an injector. Such thoughts, however, were quickly dismissed. With its help, mornings passed without incident and I could join the family at breakfast.

5 ✦ DENIAL

It took a long time for us to understand the impact of diabetes, and a longer time still to sit down and talk about it. Perhaps we didn't know what to say; perhaps we didn't want to draw attention to something we could neither accept nor change. From the outset, it seemed the only honorable course of action was to keep a stiff upper lip and take it all in stride.

"I learned from your mother over the telephone that diabetes was not curable, but that you could lead a normal life," my father said to me, recalling his first brush with diabetes. "The standard thing they put out about diabetes is just what we were told. They told us diabetes is controllable, and that you were a diabetic for life. I was relieved to learn that you really were all right, that there wasn't an emergency, and that it didn't seem logical for me to come back at that time from the mountains.

"It was an entirely clinical approach, and it still surprises me that in all of my early contact with diabetes books and doctors there was nothing as to how to handle you psychologically, or how to handle myself psychologically.

"But I guess it all pointed in a positive way. That with control you can lead a normal life. And I think I bought that hook, line, and sinker. I didn't question that control wasn't possible."

Living with disease, however, isn't a matter of logic alone. The laws of medicine work through the character of people. As people are unique, so is their relationship to and their understanding of disease. Diabetes never neatly conformed to intellectual understandings. We needed to balance the way we thought life should be with the reality of a disease that couldn't be cured and wouldn't stand still. The variables of insulin, diet, exercise, schedules, emotions, and season could gang up and bring uncertainty into our lives that we didn't know how to handle. To keep ahead of our fears, we held on to the appearance of strength. Diabetes forced a courageous strategy and a powerful determination that nothing should, nothing would forestall my growth and dreams. We proceeded with what we thought character might be, regardless of the hidden cost. We were as brave as we knew how to be, and from the beginning built a faith that denied us.

It took several weeks just to come face to face with diabetes for the first time. My mother and I were in Dr. Holland's office just before I left the hospital, and he was talking to us about the urine tests. He emphasized the importance of measuring exactly five drops of urine and ten drops of water to obtain the correct results. My mother assured the good Dr. Holland that she understood.

"How often will we have to do this?" she asked.

"Five times a day," he answered.

"Fine," she replied. No problem, she thought. There was a small bottle of tablets that came with the kit. It held maybe thirty.

"Will these be enough?" she asked. "How long do we have to do this?" Dr. Holland looked at her and suddenly saw she didn't understand. Somehow she still thought the tests would be over in four or five days.

"Mrs. Pray," he said gently, "he needs to take these tests for the rest of his life." It wasn't until then that she realized my having been in the hospital for a week really wasn't going to do it, and that nothing was going to do it. Diabetes was for a lifetime, and it was suddenly a staggering thought.

"We were up to going all out in taking perfect care of you for a month or so, but not a lifetime," she said, thinking back on it. "That was really going to affect us.

"Actually, the treatment of diabetes was rather frightening. At the hospital they taught me how to get the proper dosage, how to give you shots, what would happen if there were too much or too little, what to expect if it was insulin shock or how the opposite was diabetic coma. The two extremes resulted in not very neat things, and it looked to me as though it was going to be practically impossible.

"So in some ways I was terrified to bring you home. The only thing I can compare it to is the feeling I had just before bringing you home from the hospital as a baby. I remember that feeling when it hit me that all the hospital's support systems would be gone, that all the props would be suddenly taken away and it was up to me alone to nurture and support this new baby.

"That's how I felt when you were ready to come home from the hospital in Rumford. All those nurses that had been giving you shots, keeping you on your diet, and doing all of those things would be gone, and I knew that diabetes would be for a lifetime. I was nervous about the long cross-country trip we had ahead of us, but mostly I realized we had a lifetime trip ahead of us."

But none of this filtered its way through to me. If there were thoughts of fear or resentment, guilt or uncertainty, they were buried beneath the reassuring warmth of my hospital room.

"Did you sense my nervousness back then?" she asked.

"No," I answered.

"I would come into your room and I didn't want to dwell on the negatives. I wanted you to think everything was really okay, that your life was not ruined, and that everything was going to be just the same as it was."

"That's the feeling I had," I said. "There wasn't any fear. I only remember the warm room and the peaceful feeling of you sitting by my side."

Diabetes was an adventure, and my mother was my first and most steadfast companion. I didn't know that she was in search of other diabetic families with whom she could talk, how pleased and reassured she was to find a diabetic boy at the lake who told her he had "no problem whatsoever" giving himself the shots. I didn't know that she sat quietly in part to keep her uncertainties from spilling over onto me. Neither of us really knew what diabetes was, but we silently determined to meet it head on. Any fears we had would be kept to ourselves. It was something we shared, something we would always keep in mind, but it wasn't something we could talk about.

34

Dick Evans came over to our house for dinner one night and we talked about those early years of diabetes. I told him about our courage in the face of uncertainty. Dick admired my family. He felt drawn to our enthusiasm, to our resolve not to let problems get us down. Many families give up in the face of adversity. But the more we talked about it, the more he saw our Achilles' heel. No family is all good or all bad. No fear can be entirely denied, no matter how positive the family may seem.

He asked how we had handled the anger that must have been part and parcel of finding ourselves knee-deep in an incurable disease. I told him there wasn't any anger in the early days. Even later when there were "problems" I couldn't recall much anger. Diabetes wasn't easy, but there was nothing to be angry about.

"But how did your parents handle their anger toward you for becoming diabetic?"

"Their anger?" I asked. "I don't think anger is it." I wondered how there could have been anger when it was our strength that had carried us through all the years.

"Let me give you an example," he said. "Didn't you have a sense that you had done something bad by being diabetic? When you were at the restaurant in New Hampshire, and when you were having to sneak the water, you felt you were doing something wrong and that you were inconveniencing everybody."

"You're right," I said, "but I hadn't associated that with anger."

"Your parents must have done everything they could to convince you they didn't mind, and that they were very happy to take care of your special needs. You felt the same way. But at some level they did mind. Being human beings, they have the same selfish side to them that every human being has, and in some way that must have leaked out and you must have sensed it. I think every diabetic must feel that resentment, no matter how hard his parents try to convince themselves that they really don't resent their child.

"Did anyone ever try to help you as a family talk about the anger?"

"No," I said. "In fact, if anyone had asked me when I was eight or twelve or twenty about the anger I felt as a diabetic, I could no more have answered or even understood the question than the man in the moon. Thoughts like that just didn't go through my head.

"We tried to keep a stiff upper lip. You can't go backwards in life, and resenting it would have felt useless. We just did our best to go ahead."

"And you couldn't talk about it," said Dick.

"Talking about it would have felt like complaining."

"Why? You shared the challenges and burdens of diabetes, and yet you couldn't talk about the struggles you shared."

Finally the message began to sink in. The diabetes we had so positively accepted at the outset had been a constant and silently feared member of our family. We really couldn't talk about it beyond the specifics, beyond our hopes and determination that it wouldn't get in the way. It wasn't until I was eventually married and had three children of my own that we could even sit down and begin to share our stories. With the best intentions in the world, we kept our fears to ourselves. We believed diabetes should never become an excuse or a problem and worked double time to make sure it didn't. Our positive approach overshadowed the concerns and strengths we needed to share. The focus became our handling of diabetes rather than the hard-learned lessons that diabetes would eventually teach us.

"Part of the truth is that your parents resented having to take care of you, and you must have resented them for having passed the need on to you. At even an early age, kids hold their parents responsible for things like that.

"A lot of diabetics and their families feel the same way you did. And their families often seek to conceal the fear. Many don't ever get over it. So much depends on the message they get from their parents and how much it is explained to them what's going on. It depends on how much they realize it isn't their fault. But that is far easier said than done. There are diabetics who feel they've become diabetic because they did something wrong. Learning to accept diabetes is no easy matter."

Acceptance was to be the battle I'd fight but wouldn't understand until the battle was over. It began slowly, but as I aged the conflicts and denials would gather a terrific intensity and become a central issue in my life. From that first summer night in New Hampshire, character became synonymous with keeping ahead of the uncertainties of the disease. For my father, my mother, and me, this was all to be kept behind the scenes.

"Are most of your experiences since that summer connected with diabetic controls?" my father asked when we eventually shared our stories.

"Yes," I said. "And I think that's why there aren't many experiences I remember before becoming diabetic."

"Really?" he said with careful and almost apprehensive surprise. "Do you mean that diabetes is an ever-present, really major force in your life? It isn't something you can put on the shelf?"

"No," I said, "the undercurrents are always there." There was a pause between us, a recognition of something neither of us had ever fully acknowledged with each other.

"And as the mother of a diabetic," said my mother, "it was exactly the same way for me. I never, ever was without thinking about it. And either in a caring way, or in just planning out when the meals would come, what they would be composed of, how you were doing in school, what was going to be there when you came home from school, I think the care of you was just paramount all of the time. And I never really shed myself of that."

6 • DISCOVERIES

Aside from my family and third-grade teacher, few people knew I was diabetic. I personally told nobody, figuring my parents would tell anyone who really needed to know. As far as I was concerned, not that many people really needed to know. There were more important things to be concerned about. The mere transition from printing to cursive writing struck me as a momentous and exciting initiation into the adult world. They write the way writing should be, I said to myself as I tried to beat the class by slipping script letters into our last few printing exercises.

Anything that smacked of the ideal caught my attention and focused my energies. Diabetes itself was part of that ideal world where life went according to plan as long as I kept trying. The approach carried over from diabetes into field trips. One day we wrote letters to our parents before taking a field trip to the post office. Mrs. Millice had told us to make absolutely certain to stick the stamp at the upper right-hand corner of each envelope. She said "right" as though she really meant it, and I spent the entire morning wondering what would happen if by some accident I made a mistake. I felt for my heart at least fifty times, and then compared my upper right-hand corner with the upper right-hand corners chosen by my classmates. They seemed to have no problem distinguishing right from left. But I was sure that no matter how hard I tried, my stamp would end up on the wrong side. I imagined the entire post office grinding to a halt as the postmaster singled me out as the one kid who couldn't tell right from left. But when I handed him my letter, he took it like everybody else's and popped it into the cancellation machine. Much to my relief, it even arrived home the next day.

I didn't make friends easily, even when I had the chance. Other kids always seemed so different. I didn't pin it on diabetes, but they always had a casual attitude toward each other that would never have worked for me. I loved to compete, but the give-and-take of competition felt unnatural. In the afternoons kids would hang around carom tables on the playground. The object was to take a cue and shoot small wooden circles into the board's side pockets. Somehow I became quite good and loved nothing better than to be considered something of a newcomer and then beat everyone in sight. That, however, happened only if I was one of the first ones at the table. If a crowd arrived before me, I'd take a look and begin to walk home. Carom contacts didn't become friends. Whereas most kids were playing war games, bragging about what their fathers had done during the war, and playing Cowboys and Indians, I was more concerned about who got shot and what had happened to the Indians.

To me the Indians represented something orderly, wise, sound, and secure. They had a quality I admired and wanted to share. If I could have been an Indian before the white men came, it would have been wonderful. The fact that I would have died of diabetes never crossed my mind. Relatives gave me Indian books for Christmas, and I ended up lecturing the class on how to build a hogan.

One afternoon after classes, Holling Clancy Holling, who had written many of the books I'd read about Indians, came to our school auditorium with a replica of the canoe named *Paddle-to-the-Sea*. *Paddle* was the story of a small canoe that was carved one winter by an Indian boy and placed on a mountain slope north of Lake Superior. With the spring melt-off, *Paddle* moved down the mountain and into the rivers of the north country. The book traced *Paddle*'s self-assured voyage through the forests, across the five Great Lakes, and on into the Atlantic. Despite forest fires, shipwrecks, Niagara Falls, and the desires of his finders, *Paddle* never lost sight of his purpose. Nothing could stop him; nothing could get in his way. I knew every passage, every picture from the spellbinding book by heart.

Believing the story was true, I didn't want to meet Mr. Holling and find out it might be only a story. After he spoke, my mother urged me to meet Mr. Holling and see the canoe he brought with him for myself. I didn't want to go, but there was no saying no. When she moved forward, I reluctantly followed. I finally asked him if the small canoe he held in his hand was the actual *Paddle-to-the-Sea* that had made the great voyage. He looked somewhat surprised, and then glanced at my mother as if to learn how to answer. I knew in an instant the story wasn't true. But it didn't matter, and I determined to hold on to the vision that the Indian boy and his courageous canoe had touched within me.

Every once in a while, despite my control and determination that diabetes wasn't much of a problem, reality would pop up in an unforgettable way. One night we held a pot-luck supper at our house. Everyone brought some kind of salad or main dish, and my mother arranged the food around the kitchen table. The guests mingled between the kitchen and living room, chatting quietly and seeming to enjoy themselves. When the dinner hour came, they kept talking, and I began to feel my hunger spread into the shakiness of a reaction. I knew I was supposed to eat at six o'clock sharp, and the kitchen clock now read 6:15. I went over to my mother and asked her if the kids couldn't start and she gave us the okay.

We gathered our plates and headed for the salad table. There were all kinds of salads to choose from, and all of them looked good. I saw one of pineapple mixed with small white speckles that looked something like cottage cheese. I took several large spoonfuls, thinking that the fruit would fit right in with my diet.

With the first bite I knew something was wrong. It had an entirely foreign taste. It wasn't bitter, salty, or sour. The pineapple was masked by something almost repulsive. I tried one more bite to make sure, and it tasted the same. It was no good. Maybe something was wrong with the salad. I went to my mother.

"What is this?" I asked.

"What do you mean?" she said. A worried look crossed her face for just a second. She peered into the salad on my plate and then at the salad on the table.

"What is the white stuff?" I asked again. She tasted it.

"Larry," she said with a sense of concern and relief, "it's marshmallow. You shouldn't eat it. It's too sweet."

"Oh," I said, putting down the plate, "it tasted terrible." By now there were several people standing around the salad table.

"You know what?" she said with affection. "Your taste has completely changed. You have eaten so few sweets that they taste terrible to you. Isn't that something?" The people around us marveled at the thought, and I was surprised myself at the change.

I thought of the time I had eaten watermelon pickle at my grandfather's house when we returned from Maine to California. It had looked so good sitting in the cut-glass dish that I had already taken several delicious pieces when a cousin asked if it wasn't too sweet for me. We consulted the books the hospital had given us and discovered that watermelon pickle was cured with sugar and therefore should be avoided. I ate no more. But this time the same sweet taste felt foreign and almost disgusting.

We continued to talk for a few moments about what a remarkable and healthy change it was. When the adults moved back to the living room, I went to the table and chose another kind of salad. But as I took some of the tossed greens, the mark of distinction turned into another quiet gulf between me and the other kids at the table. They ate pineapple with marshmallow and I ate the greens. While I appreciated the distinction, I felt again that the difference was greater than met the eye.

It wasn't long after that the thought of cheating crossed my mind for the first time. It grew slowly and gradually. A small five-and-dime store stood just across the street from our school. Walking home from caroms and class each afternoon, I could see the notebooks, pencils, racks of chips and gum, candy bars and soft drinks.

My first instinct was to keep away from it. After all, I already had all the school supplies I needed, and I didn't eat candy. Besides, I was diabetic and if I went in I would stick out like a sore thumb. Everyone knew that diabetics shouldn't eat candy, and everyone would obviously know I was diabetic. Nobody had really told me why I couldn't eat candy, but the message came through loud and clear. Candy was at the top of the forbidden-foods list. But none of this cut my curiosity to find out what would happen if, despite all my misgivings and all the cardinal rules of diabetes, I went into that store and asked for a candy bar just as all the other kids did.

It took me weeks to decide it was worth a try. Rationalizing the attempt would have been easy. I'd been told many times that if I ever felt shaky or hungry it would be fine to grab a candy bar if I'd run out of Life Savers. But whom was I kidding? I didn't need a candy bar, I simply wanted to see what would happen if I ate one. I wanted to cheat. And I was scared to death to try.

After thinking about it from the school side of the street one afternoon, I gathered all my courage and went across. Looking down, I pushed the swinging screen door and entered the store. There were lots of kids inside, and it was crammed with every conceivable kind of treat. As I remember it, the elderly lady behind the counter wore a black dress. If it wasn't black, it should have been. To me she was the keeper of Snow White's candied apples, of candy bars, and of all the things a diabetic shouldn't have.

Feeling as though everyone were watching me, I edged up to the counter and tried to look nonchalant. The kid in front of me casually asked the lady for some gum and handed over his money, and she gave it to him with no questions asked. I was next in line and saw in a flash what might happen.

"What are you doing here?" she would ask with a suspicious voice.

"I'd like a candy bar, please."

"What did you say?" she'd say, looking at me very carefully. "Say that again," she'd say, suspecting the worst and trying to lead me into confession.

"A Milky Way," I'd reply with a fading voice, almost forgetting to add the "please."

"Don't you know," she would say, leaning over the counter to nail me at eye level, "that you can't have a candy bar?" By now all the kids in the store would have stopped reading their comic books to watch me.

"You are," she would say with disdain, "a diabetic." The word "diabetic" would catch the attention of every kid in the store. Even those outside on the porch would be listening intently. "And we all know," she'd say, staring me straight in the eye, "that diabetics are not supposed to have candy."

"But," I'd try to say—but it would be useless, as I would be caught dead to rights. I'd be a cheater, a liar, and a diabetic.

But that is not what happened. The kid in front of me paid for his gum with the greatest of ease, and as soon as she dropped his nickel in the cash box she looked calmly at me.

"I'd like a Milky Way," I said, holding out my nickel. I'd rehearsed that line for several weeks, and it worked perfectly. She took my nickel, reached into the glass case, and lifted out the brown candy bar with green-and-white MILKY WAY letters. She handed it to me and I took it. And that was the end of that.

Stunned with my success, I quickly walked out of the store and crossed to the other side of the street. I kept the Milky Way bar in my pocket for at least two blocks. Every so often I'd reach in and move it around in the palm of my hand. Finally I pulled it out and unwrapped it. It seemed so definite, so well made. So perfect. I bit into it, and ate it.

By the time I got home, I felt sick. Whether it was from a surge of sugar or a surge of guilt I'll never know. I walked through the door, went into my room, and lay down. My mother asked me what the matter was, perhaps instinctively knowing something wasn't right. I told her I wasn't feeling well. But I never told her about the Milky Way bar, and it was the last one I bought for many years.

7 ✦ HISTORY AND MECHANICS

It took me several years to gain a personal understanding of diabetes and its history. Like most educations that one doesn't forget, it didn't come from long talks with my parents or doctors. It was a blend of my growing experience with the disease, fragments of conversations, and my exploration of adult books about diabetes.

The books were kept on a shelf somewhat beyond reach near my parents' bedroom. I'd reach for them only when nobody else was around, noting precisely where they stood on the shelf, and then read them standing up for fear of being caught. It didn't make much sense, but reading those books felt like trespassing. In fact, my parents would probably have been glad to see me reading any one of the guides to diabetes. Such a discovery might have provided an "opening" for the kind of discussions families often seek but seldom seem to find. We all knew the basics of diabetes, and I had no burning questions in particular. But reading the books always felt like a private matter, like a venture into an adult world, and I didn't want to be seen investigating my disease. Some of what I saw touched me deeply, some of it I scarcely understood, as I browsed through the books several times a year on empty afternoons.

Diabetes, the first few pages of each book invariably said, is not a new disease. It has been recorded by many civilizations. It was noticed by the Egyptians, studied by the Greeks and Romans, and "cured" in our own age. Before the discovery of insulin, the result, when it struck children, was death. Those children, I'd say to myself as I read through the chapters, must have found themselves with the same sensations I'd felt on the journey to Maine. Something beyond understanding was happening to them, and there was nothing they could do to stop it. They were disconnected from themselves and others, and they couldn't get through. They too were thirsty, hungry, and tired. Their food no longer nourished, and what they drank never quenched their thirst. Their sweet and pale urine attracted flies and dogs. It was as though they were being purged. The more they lost their strength, the more they lost their spirit. They couldn't keep up. In the end, they must have fallen into a sleep, just as I had on the way to Rumford. There was only one difference between us: I woke up, and they continued their sleep.

I imagined their parents looking on with a sense of helplessness. Even as late as 1920 there was little they could do. Perhaps the process could be delayed by starvation diets, but the slide was inevitable. Diabetes struck adults more frequently than children, but it was on children and adolescents that it took the greater toll. With them I felt a strange kinship that grew stronger with the years. We had shared an experience. I returned and they didn't, but we were the same.

Diabetes, the books generally said, was an inherited disease. Two diabetics would most certainly have a diabetic baby, and it was slightly more common in girls than in boys. Some thought that juvenile-onset and adult-onset diabetes were separate diseases. Charts with X's and Y's traced the chances of inheriting diabetes. Its presence in cousins or grandparents greatly increased the odds. This part of the book didn't fit in my case, because I was the first one in the family to become a juvenile diabetic. Whenever a doctor asked if diabetes ran in either side of my family, I'd proudly tell him no, I was the first one to have it, and that it had just come "out of the blue." It felt good not to be a run-of-the-mill diabetic who had inherited the disease from his mother or father directly. It wasn't until years later that I learned about the strange and distant cousin named Tweet who had died of diabetes as a teen-ager before the discovery of insulin. But even then, I smugly said to myself, Tweet was a *distant* cousin many times removed, and in my own mind I remained an exception. Still later I would learn that the books were wrong, and that diabetes might be caused by a virus and only the vulnerability to the virus might be inherited.

One book showed two pictures of a young diabetic man. The first was taken just before the discovery of insulin. He looked gaunt, emaciated, and tired. The picture felt as though it had been taken for the texts of death and disease. It reminded me of the few but unforgettable pictures I'd seen of concentration-camp prisoners. This man too was trapped by something almost beyond understanding. But the second picture showed the same man with a new life. This picture had been taken shortly after he had received insulin, and the difference was miraculous. He had regained his spirit and had filled out his frame, and his expression was one of hope. The striking difference was beyond belief.

It was to the credit of Drs. Frederick G. Banting and Charles H. Best that this man lived, and that I could stand there with the book in my hand. Their names became household words to all of us very early in the game. Dr. Banting, who had a rather thin frame himself, and his student helper, Charles Best, performed their quiet experiments at a small laboratory in Canada. It had been learned in the eighteen hundreds that the pancreas, which was a word I learned long before my classmates, was directly connected with diabetes. It was a simple matter of cause and effect. If a dog's pancreas was removed, the dog developed diabetes. Everyone knew the pancreas secreted digestive juices, but no one knew exactly how it related to diabetes. The most obvious experiments didn't help answer the question. When pancreases were ground up and given to diabetic animals, the animals invariably died.

Banting and Best tried a new approach, thinking that perhaps the digestive juices in the pancreas might be destroying some magic ingredient before it could be isolated. Their hunch proved right. After eliminating the destructive digestive juices, they discovered a hormone called insulin. Although present in only minute amounts, perhaps it was the key.

Their experiments had been conducted on a group of laboratory dogs. They had extracted the dogs' pancreases to discover insulin.

Needless to say, the dogs quickly became diabetic. Now they needed only to reintroduce the hormone and wait for the results. I loved to read about the affection that grew between the doctors and their dogs in the small Toronto lab. Each dog became a pet and personality. If one died in the course of their experiments, it was considered a loss in personal as well as scientific terms. The insulin had to work, not only for the diabetics, but for their patient and trusting dogs as well.

It worked. The dogs responded to the injections as if by magic. Sadly, those who received no injections died. The key had been found, and the only next step was to try it on a human being. Although the gap from man to dog seemed somewhat large, there was really very little to lose. If the insulin didn't work, the man would die. If it did work, he would be saved. He had nothing to lose and a world to gain. Dr. Banting found a patient on the brink of death, the very patient pictured in the book. His name was Leonard Thompson. It was January 11, 1922, and once again it worked.

Word of the discovery spread rapidly throughout the world, hailing insulin as a cure for diabetes. Banting and Best were not the only doctors working on a cure for diabetes. Others were also in the process of discovering new and complicated things about digestion, the pancreas, and diabetes. Many of them had bigger names and grander reputations than Dr. Banting and Dr. Best, which served to turn both of them into heroes in my eyes. Their work received the Nobel prize, though some researchers were jealous of the victory. To me the good doctors had heroic character, and I determined that if I ever became a doctor I would be like Dr. Banting.

It is ironic that the new "cure" later became a problem. Although Dr. Banting knew better, insulin was widely viewed as the ultimate cure for diabetes. It was to diabetes what the Salk vaccine was to be to polio. There was no talk of complications, no talk of insulin as a temporary stopgap measure until a genuine cure could be found. Research continued here and there, but on a diminished basis. New suspensions and crystals of insulin were developed; the Isles of Langerhans, which produced the insulin itself, and other parts of the pancreas that I read about but rarely understood became better known and documented. But the bulk of the work was over, and in everyone's mind, including mine, diabetes had its cure. It would take a massive advertising and public-relations blitz, labeling diabetes as the third major killer behind cancer and heart disease, to break the perception that insulin was a cure.

I eventually learned how insulin worked, and came to understand the difference between my artificial shots and the way it should be if diabetes could ever be cured. When normal people ate food (later to be known as carbohydrates, proteins, and fats), it was digested, turned into sugar, and transported through the blood to the cells within the body. Insulin transformed sugar into energy. Without insulin, the sugar stayed in the blood with nowhere to go. Without insulin, cells could not receive the energy and nourishment they needed to survive.

In a normal person, the body produced insulin on demand. When a big meal produced lots of sugar, the pancreas, which I had been told looked like a bunch of squished-together grapes, produced just the right amount of insulin. If someone skipped a meal, it produced very little insulin. Every normal person's pancreas responded to the ebbs and flows of daily life. There was no waiting, no excess, no error.

But the pancreas of a diabetic didn't work. I imagined that mine had more or less shriveled up and disappeared. If any of it still remained, I told myself, it probably looked like a cluster of dry and shriveled-up raisins. The picture was inaccurate, but the result was the same. When I ate a meal, no insulin was secreted. Food still turned into sugar, but then it had nowhere to go. My body would try desperately to get rid of the excess by passing it off through my urine. The more sugar, the more water was needed to flush it from my system. Unable to derive energy from the sugar, my body turned to its internal stores of nourishment and broke down reserves of fat and muscle protein. But when fat cells are metabolized without insulin, the byproducts are poisons called ketones. These too spill off through the urine. As my body kept struggling for strength and broke down more and more fats, more and more ketones accumulated. Eventually, the process would result in coma and death. I began to understand why I had lost so much weight and why my thirst had been insatiable that summer at Pine Hill.

But Banting's discovery of insulin changed all that. With the addition of insulin, my body could get back to work. The thought of

48

staying alive with an extract of beef and pork pancreases didn't bother me in the least. The small vials of cloudy NPH looked clean and scientific, and didn't give the slightest hint of a slaughterhouse. Hopefully there would always be an ample supply of beef and pork, and the Lilly Company would never lose interest in making insulin. I was thankful it worked.

However, there were a few hitches thrown into the scheme of things. Whereas a normal person's insulin worked on demand, mine couldn't. Once injected each morning, it was there for keeps. And whereas a normal person's insulin didn't need four or five hours of lead time to reach effectiveness, mine did. NPH had its own timetable and worked independently of whatever I did. No pancreas controlled its operation. It peaked and faded at certain times of the day. Because the peaks and valleys rarely coincided with mealtimes or the schedule of my day, the trick was to give it ample (but never too much) sugar to burn. Balancing the needs of insulin with my diet (and vice versa) was the name of the game.

When NPH came on strong in the late afternoon, I'd feel myself begin to walk on the thin ice of a potential reaction as it swung into full force. If there wasn't enough food for the insulin to burn, it would search for fuel in my liver and muscles and begin to short-circuit my nervous system. I'd begin to feel shaky, nervous. My perceptions would become sharper than normal, my eyes wouldn't focus, and bright lights would blind me. It could happen all at once or snowball until I ate some food or until it found enough hidden reserves within me to quell the reaction.

In the early years the reactions were subtle. Later on their workings became violent. Without care, insulin could be a fire in search of anything to burn. In fact, taking my morning shot reminded me of lighting a small fire and waiting for it to flare later in the day. Usually it burned under control, but any error could fan the flames into a forest fire. The key was to take just the right amount. Too much insulin and I'd end up in a reaction. Too little and the opposite would happen: The injected insulin would be overwhelmed in a landslide of sugar from too big a meal. I'd then become sleepy and sick to my stomach. My kidneys would attack the problem head on, and I'd urinate as I had in Maine, and feel the same useless thirst return.

I learned, but often confused, the technical names of the two extremes. Too much sugar was called hyperglycemia. Although it took time to gather momentum, running high could eventually result in death. Too much insulin and not enough sugar was called hypoglycemia, nicknamed a reaction. It could strike like lightning; but running low could be averted with a candy bar. While I could never get the names straight, the remedies I never forgot. If I became shaky, I needed sugar in a hurry. When I felt my blood suffocate with sugar it couldn't use, I needed insulin. It was as simple as that.

There were, however, a few additional factors that had to be taken into account. Exercise required sugar. The more I exercised, the more sugar I'd need. That meant that a lot of exercise and a normal amount of food could lead me into a reaction. Whenever my father and I took hikes through the San Gabriel Mountains, which rose north of our home, we'd carry rolls of the aptly named Life Savers. I couldn't leave home without them. On the other side of the coin, if there passed a day when I didn't exercise at all, there would be too much sugar. The trick, once again, was to achieve a fine balance and then keep it day in and day out.

Each book stressed that diet was the key to successful diabetes management, and so it was. An insulin dose could be controlled only at the time of injection, whereas the amount of food could be controlled throughout the day. Depending on the circumstances, I could make adjustments as needed. But I had to be careful and know what I was doing. If I ate too much or too little, it would mean trouble one way or the other. Even a small excess or a forgotten glass of breakfast juice could throw things off kilter. To keep everything regulated, all food was measured in calories and exchanges. Although we kept a chart taped to the refrigerator, we rarely needed it. My mother and I knew all the exchanges by heart. We knew exactly how many were to be taken at each meal or snack, and the foods that constituted each exchange.

Thirty grams of meat, for example, was one meat exchange. So was one medium egg. Half a glass of juice provided the same number of calories as one medium apple, three small prunes, or half a banana. A measly 15 grams of raisins were the equivalent of half a grapefruit or a whopping 175 grams of watermelon. Needless to say, watermelon fast became a favorite. One slice of bread, one bowl of cereal, one-half a small ear of corn and five saltines were all the same: one bread exchange. I could eat a larger bowl of Puffed Rice than of Grape Nuts, but the cereal in each had to weigh the same 20 grams. Carrots were to be eaten in moderation, but celery and cabbage were more or less on the house. Some foods went to work immediately; others took longer to release their energy. Each meal needed a balance of both. Our job was to make sure the injected insulin had just the right amount of fuel to consume at all times, and to balance it with the correct amount of exercise.

To keep track of things, we used the urine tests Dr. Holland had prescribed back in Maine. Known as "Clinitests," they indicated when something was off and which way to turn. I loved the vindication of a deep blue test, and hated watching the bright orange settle out in the test tube to show I wasn't doing something right. In either case, exact records had to be kept at all times.

Cheating would have been possible. Fifteen drops of water without any urine always produced a blue test. But the solution didn't look the same. It was too thin, the blue too light. Besides, the idea of cheating didn't seriously cross my mind. The tests were important, and no true student of science would interfere with the wonders of chemistry. Thinking my newfound sense of chemical expertise might have some applications, I tried at one point to do my own Banting and Best experiment by testing the urine of a frog.

According to the Clinitest label, it was vital to carefully follow the instructions to obtain correct results. I wrote the Ames Company and asked if two drops of water and one minute drop of frog urine would work if I used one-fifth of a Clinitest tablet. Several weeks later they wrote back. They knew of somebody working on diabetes in animals, and included a copy of some man's research. His treatise said nothing about testing the urine of a diabetic frog, but it looked very complicated and scientific. They thanked me for my letter, and I must say I was duly impressed.

The tests were the one part of diabetes I wasn't afraid to show off. They gave me an "in" to privileged information that other kids just didn't have. Just before we left California and near my ninth birthday, a distant cousin was showing me his new chemistry kit, complete with all kinds of colorful chemicals. It was most impressive, but

I decided to show him one better. I went out to the car and brought in my Clinitest kit. Once it was set up on the counter and the POISON label on the jar of tablets had been seen by everyone, including his sisters, I asked for directions to the bathroom. In a minute or two, I returned with an eyedropper full of urine. Everyone gathered around to watch the great experiment.

The five drops of yellow liquid found their way into the glass test tube. We rinsed out the eyedropper several times and then added ten precise drops of water. With great fanfare, I dropped in the blue-and-white-speckled tablet and we all watched it froth into a delightful blue. Everyone was impressed, especially my cousin the chemist. But his sisters began giggling and left the room. Once they were gone, he quietly told me they knew what was in the eyedropper and that was why they were giggling. I was shocked. How could they possibly have known? How could they laugh at my chemistry? Was it the same for girls too? And wasn't the whole test a secret that only diabetics understood? I was crushed. Needless to say, it was the last time I tested in public, and the last time I ever told anybody I tested.

In any event, these were the mechanics, and I knew they counted. As I put the books back on their shelves at the same exact angle as I'd found them, I'd wonder about the connection between me and all that I'd read. It applied directly, but then again, it didn't. The descriptions were accurate, but I would close the book as though they didn't really pertain to me. That was the paradox. The books were at once true and false, helpful in understanding the mechanics of diabetes and hopeless in bridging the gap between me and my disease. We had, after all, been given two sets of prescriptions from our first days at the hospital. The first read: "THE REQUIREMENTS AND RESTRICTIONS OF DIABETES MUST BE MAINTAINED WITHOUT FAIL." The second, and perhaps more powerful, read: "As a diabetic, you can lead a perfectly normal life."

8 · CAMP

Part of being normal meant going to camp. My parents thought it would be a good idea for me to meet other diabetic kids, to have some new experiences, and to see that diabetes was not a limiting disease. Just as I had begun to take my own shots right off the bat, so I went to camp the summer following my diagnosis.

The Milwaukee Boys Club ran a camp that blended diabetic and nondiabetic kids. We had all decided that attending a camp with only diabetic kids would be overly therapeutic, and quickly dismissed the idea. The last thing we wanted was to separate me from the mainstream of life. Camp Whitcomb seemed to fill our every need.

As with most summer camps, its brochure talked about a beautiful lake, gave a vivid description of the fine facilities and healthful programs, and included some color postcards of the totem poles at the camp's entrance. This camp specialized in Indian lore, and I was sure I'd like it. It would also be my first extended sojourn away from home and relatives as a diabetic. It was a big step for all of us, and everyone was sure I could handle it.

Once I'd been dropped off, however, I thought the two weeks would never end. There were no near reactions, no candy bars, and no near misses during my entire stay, but camp threw me into a world I wasn't sure I wanted. I'd avoided making friends before, but now I had to make friends to get along. I now needed to join the groups that I'd always seen from a distance. And I had to reconcile the comforting world of home and confidence with the ghost stories of camp.

Night after night I tried to hide my head under the pillow as our counselor told us frightful stories that had to be true. From time to time I'd throw out a "Wow!" or an "Oh, geeze!" to sound convincing, and then retreat to whatever silence I could find. But the sound of the stories came through no matter what I did. When he told about the green slime that had begun, on an August night many years before, to ooze out of the lake and work its way up past the dining hall and on into the cabins, I knew there was no way to keep it out.

One night all the new campers were told to stand in a circle around a blazing bonfire. An Indian chief, who had appeared magically right out of the woods, told us to repeat an old and sacred chant that sounded something like Ohwah Tagoo Siam. He told us to continue chanting and bowing until the sacred message of old revealed itself to us. We said it over and over ever so seriously and waited for the Great Spirit to convey the hidden meaning. After a while I noticed that many kids, both diabetic and nondiabetic, were getting the message before me. They'd suddenly stop bowing, begin to laugh, go up to the chief, whisper to him the secret message, and sit down with a big smile.

But try as I might, no such message came through. I kept trying harder and harder to do it right, to follow the instructions of the chief. After a while, there were only about three of us left standing there in front of the entire camp saying with equal measures of fear and embarrassment, "Oh, what a goose I am." Finally, a kindly counselor came over and personally delivered the message of the Great Spirit. I was crushed. I'd been deceived. I thought it was for real. How could they do something like that?

And I was homesick beyond belief. I was all right as long as I was working on a project or taking nature walks looking for muskrats or remnants of the green slime. And it was fine when the whole camp sang songs like "Pack Up Your Troubles in Your Old Kit Bag and Smile, Smile, Smile." I loved that song with all my heart and soul, smiled for dear life, and hoped the dinner hour would never end. But when the singing finished and everyone walked back to the cabins, the pangs of homesickness hit without fail.

54

My father visited after the first week, and I waited for him throughout the day. In the early afternoon, just when I thought he had forgotten all about me, he came walking across a small field with a fellow geologist. I have never been as glad or as moved to see someone again in my entire life. My eyes filled with tears as I ran forward to give him a hug and tried to disguise my feelings. It wasn't right to be homesick, but wasn't I glad to see him! Having the uncanny ability of most parents to see right through their children, he knew how I felt. But having the same uncanny ability children have to see right through their parents, I could tell he was surprised. He hadn't expected to find me homesick, and I could never tell him how much I'd missed him. He greeted me with an affectionate "Hi, fellah" and asked how everything was going. I told him it was just fine, and showed him around the camp until he had to leave.

Just as my father and I found it difficult to share the feelings that touched us most deeply, so it was with the kids in my cabin. We went through our days together, but never once talked about diabetes. We took our shots in the morning, checked each other's urine charts, measured our helpings at mealtime, and asked each other, the first time we met, how long we'd had the disease. But that was as far as it went. Questions like "How do you handle your diabetes?" or "Do you cheat?" or "How do you feel about being diabetic?" not only never came up, they would have felt entirely out of place if someone had made the mistake of asking. Perhaps those questions and the benefits of going to a camp with other diabetics existed more in the minds of our parents and the camp directors. Diabetes was something we didn't want to dwell on, and so we didn't. We'd been told we could lead normal lives, and we tried to do exactly that. Not talking about diabetes was one good way to do it.

If our counselor knew anything about diabetes, he kept it to himself. Every so often he would ask if we were okay, and after resenting for a moment the intrusion into our private lives we would invariably answer yes. He told us he kept rolls of Life Savers stashed away under his bunk for emergencies, but diabetes wasn't his focus either. If he had talked about it, I doubt that any of us would have known what to say. From all anyone could tell, diabetes was the furthest thing from our minds and lives.

9 • MOVING

In the summer of 1956, we moved from Pasadena to Colorado. My father had decided to stop teaching and begin research with the Ohio Oil Company. As a geologist, he studied rocks that were millions of years old, drove slowly through road cuts for no apparent reason, and loved the outdoors. Like most kids, I had only a foggy idea of what my father actually did. When he went to work, I imagined that people lined up outside his Cal Tech office with rocks in their hands. They would marvel at the skeletons of saber-toothed tigers and other prehistoric animals that lined the long hallway, and then enter his office one at a time to ask him what kind of rock they had found. He would answer with scientific certainty, and they'd be on their way.

While he'd have to find a new string of clients, we weren't sorry to leave. The smog smarted our eyes, made us wheeze when we mowed the lawn, and covered the city like a thick dirty blanket. Sometimes the view from the top of the mountains made us wonder how we could live in such smoke. It wasn't the way it was meant to be. But Colorado, he told us after his final interview, was beautiful beyond description. And it was, but it took a little getting used to.

We arrived at a brick house on a dirt road. Most of the neighbors lived some distance away, had horses, talked with a different accent, and wore boots without showing off. Dust was everywhere, but the sky above was clear. Occasional lawns and gardens seemed to hang on by the skin of their teeth. It didn't rain very much, and then only in the afternoon. The only trees were giant cottonwoods that surrounded the small dammed-up ponds and lined the irrigation ditches and dry streams. The fruit trees that we had had around our house in California were nowhere to be found. Everything had to be planted, and plant we did. Sometimes I thought I'd end up spending my entire life pulling ragweed, watering trees, and waiting for the grass to grow.

There were kids in our neighborhood, but most of them were either older or younger than I was. I really hadn't found a friend since becoming diabetic. I didn't want others to know about my disease and dreaded having anyone go out of his way for me. A close friend might mean awkward explanations that I was reluctant to give. If I was invited over to a neighbor's house, the others would end up having a snack of cookies or ice cream and I'd have to decline. They would ask why. Not wanting to get into it, I'd say, I'm just not hungry, thank you, and try to leave it at that. But it felt like pulling the wool over their eyes, and I'd always end up more of a spectator than a friend.

One big kid next door began to train hawks in his spare time, and for a while I linked up with him. His falcon traps were made of clear fish leader tied into thousands of slipknots that surrounded a small wire cage. Inside the cage were several pigeons. The hawks would swoop down for the pigeons and get caught in the invisible loops as they tried to get away. After capture came the hooding, the feeding, the training, and then the first few flights when we never knew whether the bird would stay or take to the skies. It was intriguing, but exclusively his. He taught me, but when my mother suggested I go pay him a visit (she recognized my reticence and did her best to break it down), I'd usually find something else to do. I hadn't found a friend who could share my fantasies, who wouldn't worry about my diabetes, and with whom I could explore the world.

That isolation began to break down as I entered the fourth grade. There was a kid in our class named Miles. It was a strange name, just the way Caroll was the strange name for my brief friend in Maine. I don't remember how Miles and I ever came together. Perhaps it was the attraction of two kids who, one because of his upbringing and the other because of his health, didn't fit the usual mold. Miles had grown up in a house surrounded on all sides by prairie. He and his brothers herded sheep as part of their chores, drank fresh goat's milk, lived in a house built by his father from lodgepole pine, and knew all about Colorado.

When I went home with him after school, we'd spend the afternoon walking through the pasture below his house scaring prairie dogs, chasing sheep, and waiting for trains to come and flatten the coins we'd left on the track. We'd squirt each other as we milked the goats, talk about Indians and rocket ships, and walk back to the house watching the grasshoppers fan out through the field ahead of us. When we looked up, we could see seventy miles south to Pikes Peak, fifty miles north to Longs Peak, and watch the afternoon clouds shade the entire front range of the Rockies.

We both knew that the Indians ate grasshoppers as part of their diet. One afternoon, as we walked back to his house, the grasshoppers seemed particularly plentiful. In fact, they were swarming in the thousands. And they were big.

"Wonder how the Indians ate them," I said.

"Dunno," said Miles.

"Well," I said, "I'll give you a quarter if you'll try one."

"Sure thing," replied Miles. We stopped our walk, and I caught the biggest yellow-bellied grasshopper I could find. It must have been three inches long. To make it more palatable, I squeezed it, and the brown tobacco juice that all grasshoppers chew oozed out of its mouth.

"All right," I said, "here you go. A quarter if you eat it."

"All right," said Miles. He twisted the head off and popped the rest of the grasshopper into his mouth. Once he'd swallowed it and once I was sure it was all the way down, he asked for his quarter. I reached into my pocket, but knew already that I didn't have one. He wasn't supposed to go through with it in the first place. There was only one honorable way out.

"Listen," I said, "suppose I eat one. Then we'd be even, right?" He agreed, and began to look for the biggest grasshopper in the entire pasture. He found it. It was huge. It spat its juice, squiggled as it lost its head and tried to get out of my fingers. For just a moment I wondered about the calories of a grasshopper. It wasn't on any exchange chart I'd ever seen, but I figured it wouldn't hurt. Even if it did, I was clearly stuck. Without a word, looking as Indian-like as possible, I put it into my mouth and took a decisive bite. I even swallowed it. The crunch wasn't so bad, but when that grasshopper got halfway down my throat the taste hit. I nearly threw up on the spot. It was so bad it almost got stuck at the halfway point. But I didn't say a word. We both knew it tasted terrible, yet neither one of us would admit it. Suddenly we broke out laughing. We'd each eaten a grasshopper, each had the other's imaginary quarter, and neither was a penny richer. The more we thought about it the more we laughed, and we slowly headed back to the house.

As our friendship grew, Miles invited me to spend a night at his house. I hadn't had much trouble with my diabetes, but this would be the first test outside of the family and outside of a camp. It meant I would have to take care of myself, and that he and his family needed to know I was diabetic. I imagine I told him on an afternoon walk that if he ever saw me pass out he should give me a candy bar, and I suppose my mother talked with his mother over the phone. It turned out she had once been a nurse, and would be glad to keep an open eye. My biggest fear was being hungry and then having to trespass into somebody else's refrigerator.

The exchange lists flew through my mind as we sat down to dinner. Did goat's milk count the same as cow's milk? How greasy was the fried chicken? And what about all the tomatoes and the home-made bread that was cut into irregular slices? The last thing I wanted was to disrupt their routine when they'd already gone out of their way to invite me. But I kept these thoughts to myself, and it all worked out just fine.

From our short talks, my weekends at his house, and the hours Miles and I spent designing spaceships, he knew I had to take shots and watch my diet. Instead of hampering our projects, diabetes almost enhanced our future plans. Our spaceships had normal engines, but were characterized by huge compartments of food. We designed milk compartments; fruit compartments; bread, meat, butter, and medical compartments. We even included a special insulin compartment. If the rest of our fourth-grade class wondered what we were doing when we proudly shared our designs (with the insulin com-

59

partment disguised) at Show and Tell, it was clearly their problem and not ours.

From all this, Miles was well aware I was diabetic. Part of the reason I loved our friendship, however, was that the diabetes never seemed to limit us or matter. I didn't have to be careful, didn't have to worry about fitting in. We were caught up in our boundless imaginations, and life would conform to us rather than the other way around. But neither of us was prepared for what happened one day in class when the possibilities and the depth of diabetes became clear for the first time.

What led up to it I don't remember. Dim recollections tell me I was sitting at my desk, aware that I was hungry and that I needed something to eat. Maybe I'd run to school that morning instead of walking. Maybe I'd switched cereals, or the juice had been too diluted. Whatever the case, I could feel the reaction coming on, and I was caught. Lunch was too far away, there was no recess break for the rest of the morning, and I needed something to eat. As the teacher spoke, I slipped my hand inside the desk and tried to find something without attracting attention. That was what I most wanted to avoid: I didn't want to attract attention. My hand moved around the books and papers inside my desk in search of a box of raisins or a roll of Life Savers. None were there. I could feel the reaction build, could see my hand shake, could feel I was in trouble. But the worse it got the more I tried to hold on. No matter what, I couldn't, wouldn't raise my hand, interrupt the teacher and have the class stop just for me. If I stood up and just walked out, everybody would ask what was going on. I made a final sweep of the desk and checked to see if anyone had noticed my search for food. No one had. And that is the last thing I remember.

My mother later told me I had passed out, fallen from my desk, and gone into convulsions. As I slumped over, my teacher must have rushed to my side, Miles must have wondered what was happening, and someone must have run to the front office. My mother received a telephone call. The message was "Mrs. Pray, your son is having convulsions. Please come down and get him." She grabbed a bottle of Karo corn syrup, ran frantically to the car, and tore down to the school. Somehow or other she gave me the sweet, sticky syrup; I was lifted into the car, and soon woke up.

I remember none of this. One thing about a serious reaction is that once you are in it you can't remember what happens. It is as though time were suspended. The blackout is both dangerous and beneficial. I never know what happens, but there is no fear. The strange part of the fourth-grade reaction is that we didn't talk much about it. My teacher said nothing to me about it, classmates said nothing to me, and I do not remember talking to my parents about it. Perhaps the class had been told not to mention it. Perhaps my parents simply resolved to help me prevent them in the future.

I do remember wrapping sugar cubes in aluminum foil and keeping a batch of them in my desk. I also remember a strengthening and deepening bond with my friend Miles. We soon became Indian blood brothers, complete with knife cuts and promises. It was strange, because he was such a pioneer and I didn't think I was. But we were friends, and diabetes didn't get in the way.

10 · THE GREAT HONEY INCIDENT

At mealtimes, diabetes enhanced our sense of family. Our evening meals were always family affairs that brought a double reward: each other's company as we shared our stories of the day and an unspoken but reassuring confidence that we had made it through the danger zone of diabetes to the safety of a meal.

NPH peaked in the late afternoons, so getting to dinner without incident required some family strategy. For me it began by calculating how fast I should ride my bike home from school, whether or not I needed to stop off at a friend's house for an emergency sandwich, or what kind of snack I should take once I arrived home. My mother, who was mistress of the kitchen and an excellent cook, also planned her afternoons around a six-o'clock deadline. She knew that the closer we came to six the closer I would be to a reaction, and that even a ten- or fifteen-minute delay could throw things off and upset the family balance.

Sometimes, however, our best-laid plans didn't work out. One afternoon the dog ate a steak marinating on the kitchen counter. Or maybe the chicken hadn't thawed. And every so often I was just hungrier than normal and needed dinner sooner than six. When the unexpected happened, alarm signals began to go off in all of us.

"When's dinner?" I'd casually ask, opening the icebox in search of some juice to appease the growing reaction.

"Not much longer," she'd say. "Are you going to be all right?"

"Sure," I'd say, looking for a glass. By now, however, she already had visions of trouble.

"Get some juice," she'd say, realizing that our plans had fallen through.

"I am," I'd say defiantly, wishing I hadn't said anything in the first place. The closer I was to a reaction, the more anger I felt and the more upset she'd be. Before long we'd have a full-fledged scene on our hands as it became obvious to everyone that we weren't going to make it to the safety and reassurance of a family dinner. If only dinner had been ready sooner, if only I had taken a better snack, if only, if only, if only . . . It was as though diabetes, which could pull us together in so many ways, could just as easily magnify the tiny failures of an entire day's plans into a single moment of confrontation.

The fights and close calls were not daily occurrences. In fact, they happened only rarely. Dinner was almost always at six, my snacks worked very well most of the time, and I could even disguise a reaction for a moment or two while the meal came out of the oven. But there were so many variables that the possibility of a problem remained in our minds until we finally sat down at the table, said grace, and began dinner.

I remember one afternoon incident in particular that revealed more than any of us wanted to see. It happened as I was searching the cupboard for a snack and spied a plastic jar of honey with a smiling bee on its side. I had never tasted honey. It didn't have an artificial substitute the way maple syrup did, and because diabetics were supposed to avoid it at all costs, my curiosity began to peak. Just around the corner my mother was in the midst of teaching a piano lesson, persistently coaching her pupil the same way she coached me.

"Try again," I heard her say patiently, and sure enough the melody began again. I looked back to the honey and listened. All I could hear was that simple right-hand exercise. I silently reached for the honey, tilted back my head, and squeezed a small whirl onto my tongue.

Just at that moment my mother walked into the kitchen.

"Larry," she said. Oh, my God, I thought. A feeling of shame ran through me. Her face was mixed with surprise and astonishment. She looked directly at me, and I, with the honey jar in my hand, looked directly at her. Neither of us knew what to say. It was as though she had seen something she had perhaps expected but never wanted to see. And she saw something I never wanted her to see, something I didn't want to recognize myself. It didn't matter that I didn't eat candy bars, didn't indulge in cake at friends' houses; that only once in a great while did I experiment with sweets. None of that made any difference. At that moment there could be no excuse, no defense, no alibi. After a second she turned around and went back to her pupil, who was going to stay with that melody until he learned it to perfection.

It took an eternity for dinner to come. At six o'clock she brought out the meal. We sat down at the table, said grace, and began to give the news of the day. I kept waiting for her to look at me and say, "Larry, what were you doing with that jar of honey this afternoon?" Then my father would look up and wait for an answer, my brothers would fall silent, and I myself would wait for an answer that probably wouldn't come.

But she never said a word. We went through the entire meal without even mentioning it. After dinner they didn't bring it up either, and while I certainly didn't take the opportunity myself, neither could I get it out of my mind that we let the incident slip.

"Why didn't you bring it up?" I asked my parents many years later.

"I knew you were cheating sometimes," said my mother, "but I really didn't want to embarrass you. I knew that you knew what you were doing, and that you could straighten it all out. I didn't want to ever scold you or make you feel bad about something."

"From my standpoint," added my father, "I was satisfied that you were in better control and better organized with your diabetes than we had any right to expect, and I was just grateful. I was really proud of the way you handled it throughout all those years."

Shattering is too strong a word, but The Great Honey Incident jarred my view of the family. We prided ourselves on meeting challenges head on, and yet that afternoon my mother and I had both looked the other way. For the first time it occurred to me that something in our family was lacking and that the truth about diabetes would be difficult or maybe even impossible to find.

It was, to say the least, an unfair perception. Had my parents brought up the incident as a matter of integrity, I might have never forgotten my hurt feelings. And yet when they ignored it, I couldn't quite forgive them. Either way, they lost. That kind of double bind, Dick Evans told me, is a trick kids invariably play on their parents. Kids want to see their parents as perfect, resent their fall in a no-win situation, and then hold it against them for a long time to come. It's all part of growing up and breaking away from the family.

There is a honey incident in the life of every diabetic family at one stage or another. Parents worry about what to do when their child cheats, and kids wonder what they'll do if they're caught. For both, there really isn't a right answer for a problem laced with worry and doubt. Only the extremes are clear. If the world stops in its tracks every time a diabetic tastes a spoonful of honey, there won't be much room for growth. On the other hand, if wholesale cheating is ignored for fear of rocking the boat, there may not develop the sense of accountability that is an essential part of growing up with diabetes. Finding a way between the two is the name of the game.

In our case, two messages came through. Assuming that my diabetes was well in hand kept us from sharing the challenges we faced for so many years. Looking back on it, I wish we could have taken the risk of asking questions that didn't have answers. At the same time, it was clear that what I did with my diabetes was up to me. Diabetes was my parents' concern, but my responsibility. And for that confidence, I'm still grateful.

11 ◆ MAGICAL THINKING

"Denial isn't all bad," said Dick Evans as we talked one evening. "After all, keeping one step ahead of oneself means keeping so busy you won't have time to slow down and face the facts."

"I recently heard of one newly diagnosed diabetic," I said, "who holds down two or three jobs and is doing excellent work at school. His mother said that when he sits down for a minute's rest, it's as though nervous butterflies run through him. Denial is helping push him into being that much better a student, busboy, and lobsterman. I've never had occasion to lobster, but it was much the same way with me."

"But when it comes to diabetes," said Dick, "denial doesn't work. It doesn't help with acceptance, and it can't make diabetes go away."

"That took a long time to find out," I said, thinking back on my attempts to keep diabetes at an arm's length.

For me the stakes began to escalate in 1958 when my parents and I looked for a diabetic camp in Colorado. To our surprise, there was none to be found. In fact, although the East and West Coasts had camps in nearly every state, the entire Great Plains and Mountain States lay empty. It didn't seem right to any of us that a diabetic kid in Colorado had to travel a thousand miles to find a camp, so we took it on ourselves to do what we could.

My father had become involved in the Diabetes Lay Association upon our arrival in Littleton, and creating a camp became one of its projects. After cajoling and convincing some reluctant "leading experts," he asked the Denver YMCA if it would allow a cabin of diabetics at its Camp Chief Ouray, near Granby, Colorado. The Y replied that if there was proper supervision, it would be glad to admit fourteen of us. Two doctors volunteered their time, and we were in business, both figuratively and literally as we went from door to door selling chocolate mints to earn our tuition. Needless to say, we never mentioned the fact that we were forbidden to taste-test our probably delicious mints.

In the midst of the enthusiasm and irony, there was only one hitch in the back of my mind. I hadn't seen it as a problem at Whitcomb, but the special provisions that had to be made for us at Ouray struck me as necessary but distasteful. The great part of being diabetic was that I could proceed with my life full steam ahead just like the rest of the world. At home, that is exactly what I tried to do. But at camp, I would be relegated to a cabin of diabetics only, and now that I was older I resented the label.

To overcome it, I determined to compete, earn whatever honors I could, and prove there was nothing a diabetic couldn't do. On my third day at camp, however, I was running across a clearing when I smacked my foot against a stump. It hurt far worse than a stubbed toe, and the pain didn't go away. The doctor took a look at it and decided we should drive into Granby to have it checked. The X rays revealed a small fracture of the metatarsal (a medical term that made the word "foot" sound terribly humdrum) and the hospital proceeded to put on a cast.

Our cabin had planned on taking a hike past some rare quicksand pits the next afternoon, and I fast made it known I was going to go despite the cast and my counselor's concern. When some kids said I'd hold them back, I told them they'd have to keep up with me instead. And besides, a cast might come in handy if we ran into a nest of rattlesnakes somewhere along the way.

I made it over the mountain and past the pits, kicking cactus and rocks and shrugging off all suggestions to take it easy. By the time we were back in camp, the plaster cast had disintegrated beyond recognition. The camp doctor looked at it; he laughed and said we should go back into town and get a new one.

The Granby nurse admired my spirit, but warned me to take better care of this second cast. Just to make sure it wouldn't get abused, she refused to give me a walking cast. When she handed me a pair of crutches with a slightly victorious look, it became a battle of wills. Nothing would hold me back. I even played soccer with the non-walking cast and stashed the crutches away as fast as I could. Needless to say, the cast crumbled in a few days. When we returned to town again, I had the victorious look and she gave in, telling me to wear a pair of stiff Sunday shoes instead.

For me it was a double victory. The casts hadn't stopped me from the camp's activities, and I had successfully proved that the fracture wasn't really an infirmity at all. It wasn't too long a step from overcoming a fractured metatarsal to overcoming diabetes.

"And with that," said Dick Evans, "magical thinking got under way."

"What's magical thinking?" I asked.

"Magical thinking is when you believe if you wish hard enough you can make the clouds disappear on a rainy day, or make the Red Sox win the pennant when they're ten games out in October. Magical thinking happens to everyone. I just heard of a baseball player who started getting a lot of hits once he started growing a beard. So he decided he was going to keep that beard for the rest of the season, as though the beard had something to do with his hitting. Another example might be the superstition some people have that their cards might change if they pick them up before they've all been dealt. Magical thinking is built into all of us. Your applying it to diabetes was almost inevitable. It isn't, however, a very good substitute for hard work in situations that are possible or for reality in situations that aren't possible," said Dick.

"Does it begin with denial?"

"Magical thinking is like denial in overdrive. It is an attempt to prove mind over matter, much as you tried to do with the cast. Whereas denial was a hope that diabetes wasn't really there in the first place, magical thinking raised the stakes in an attempt to get rid of it entirely by wishing it away."

Magical thinking would show itself in many ways over the next eight years. Sometimes it was a major event, sometimes no more than a passing thought. Before it ended on my twentieth birthday, it would test the full extent of my emotional and physical limits.

My first attempt at magical thinking had been a great success, and I wore my Sunday shoes like badges of invulnerability. The success, however, was short-lived. One of the diabetics in our cabin was a black kid from Houston, Texas. We were about the same age, but he seemed worlds more mature than I. As we were talking one afternoon, he caught sight of my shoes.

"Look at those shoes," he said with a smile that was creeping into a laugh. I looked down. Not only did they suddenly look out of place, they were a mess. He pointed to his shoes beside his bed. They were immaculate.

"What's wrong with my shoes?" I asked defensively.

"Don't you have any sole shine?" he asked.

"Any what?"

"Sole shine. Look at the sides of those soles. When's the last time you shined them?"

"The sides of my soles?"

"Do you mean to say you don't use sole shine?"

"You're kidding," I said.

"Kidding?" he said with a chuckle that broke into a laugh. "Where have you been all these years? In Houston nobody in their right mind would go around without the sides of their soles looking as nice as the rest."

I was incredulous. I still don't know if he was serious, and to this day look for small cans of specially developed sole shine every time I enter a shoe store. I haven't found any yet, but then, I haven't been to Houston either. That afternoon, however, the confrontation didn't make me laugh. I wasn't exactly a teasable kid, and having no intention of letting him put something over on me, I began to compete.

"Well," I said, "I just don't happen to think that shining the sides or even the top of my shoes is all that important."

"Well, well, well, listen to that," he said with an easy smile. I was flustered and embarrassed. On the surface it was a petty argument, but underneath I was practically trembling. Just then the young doctor happened along. Evidently he had heard our skirmish because he joined in and took my side.

After he left, my friend and I looked at each other, wondering what had just happened. It was as though the intensity of my emotion had caught me off guard and left me feeling bewildered, bailed out, and most of all, vulnerable. All it had taken to set me off was a tease and the easy laugh of another diabetic.

"I guess I didn't get along very well with other diabetics," I said to Dick Evans. "The few diabetics I knew at home didn't take good care of themselves and I didn't want to be like them. And the kid at camp cut right through my 'I can do anything' magical armor."

"Well," said Dick, "remember that every kid has got a pretty fragile identity. People start building their identity very early, and by the time you're an adolescent you're the most intolerant of differences in other people. Diabetes is a threat for a diabetic to grapple with in establishing his or her identity. You had the normal adjustment problems of growing up plus the added obstacle of diabetes. Getting to know other diabetics reminded you of that."

"In some ways, I envied that kid from Houston," I said. "He was diabetic, but could laugh at things so much easier than I could."

"You were trying to make things conform to your expectations," said Dick, "and that's part of magical thinking. You did that with your cast and with diabetes as a whole. Being with him tied the two of you together against your wills."

"How?" I asked.

"He was diabetic, and he threatened your identity. After all, if he was right in his approach toward life and diabetes, where would that put you?"

The question had a simple answer. If my approach was wrong, I'd be left having to face myself without much protection, and the best way to prevent that was to hang on for dear life.

"We all like to keep up a denial of our own vulnerability," continued Dick. "We do it right alongside of the knowledge we are in fact diabetic, or even when we know we are dying. In the hospital, some patients dying of cancer can't talk about it. They're afraid if they do it will destroy their ability to maintain their denial. But the wise ones talk about it freely and know they can still maintain a healthy denial. Magical thinking makes a healthy denial very difficult, because it constantly tries to change reality."

On the final night of camp, I didn't get the Outstanding Camper award. I came very close, but didn't get it. But as my heart fell when they announced somebody's else's name, another part of me suspected they had made the right decision. The other kid was more relaxed, more live-and-let-live, less caught with his head in the clouds and his feet nowhere near the ground.

12 ⋅ *CONTRADICTIONS*

Euclid Junior High School was an immense, brand-new school designed for science fairs and the space age. It was, I said to myself, time to begin preparing myself to make a mark in the world and to leave my family. After all, college was only six years down the line, competition would be tough, and my parents wouldn't always be around. In fact, my father was in Libya doing some fieldwork, and my mother had just left to join him for a trip through Europe.

It gave me a feeling of pride to know they trusted that I had my diabetes well enough in hand for them to leave. They could have assumed their presence was essential to my well-being, and that it would have been irresponsible to leave. I was glad they saw it the other way around. The trip marked part of my growing up and their letting go, and I looked forward to the test.

They hired an elderly woman named Mrs. Woods to stay with us. She wasn't the least bit intimidated by my diabetes. When she fried the green tomatoes we collected at her farm she let me take my own helpings. Unlike my mother, she would never tell me when to wear a coat, figuring I'd know when it was cold. She was right, but didn't know I'd just read a book about polar explorers who trained themselves for the Arctic through daily exposure to freezing temperatures.

Junior high was filled with those kinds of experiments. Determining who was biggest and strongest, who played the electric guitar and who didn't, falling head over heels in love (but not telling the girl or anyone else about it) occupied most of my imagination. Not knowing quite what to do with the feelings I couldn't control, I turned to areas I could control, and Scouts was one of them.

There were, thank heaven, no diabetic Scout troops. We didn't even try to look for one. For me, that was the best part of Scouting. There would be no special provisions, and only the Scoutmaster would know. He was a geologist friend of my father's, and we had an understanding that I would be more or less on my own. For all of us, Scouting became a symbol of my independence as a diabetic.

The Methodist Church sanctuary was nearly dark the night of my initiation into Troop 114. We were led to the altar and stood before a log with twelve candles in it. A Scout was to be trustworthy, an older Scout said. As he said it, the first candle was lit and a chill went up my spine. A Scout was to be loyal, helpful, friendly, courteous, kind, thrifty, obedient, cheerful, brave, clean, and reverent. Needless to say, he didn't say a Scout was diabetic. The values he had given were the epitome of excellence and transcended limitations. As I saw it, my task was to live up to those values because they represented life the way it should be.

When we received our neckerchiefs, they were brown and a turquoise shade of blue. The brown represented the bark of the ponderosa pine when wet after a thunderstorm, and the blue represented the color of the Colorado sky just before sunset turned it into stars. I stood up and shook hands with the members of my new troop. I was proud to be a Scout.

In the following weeks I learned a host of new knots and practiced them endlessly to make sure I could do them with my eyes closed at our Thursday-night meetings. I moved quickly to Second Class, six months later to First Class and began work on the merit badges that nobody else in the troop had ever earned. I spent countless hours watching the stars of the January sky, getting up at two in the morning with sky charts and a flashlight to find constellations for the Astronomy merit badge. Somehow the stars at two o'clock were more beautiful and more important than the ordinary stars of seven or eight in the evening. I was also the first to get the colorful Skiing badge, and with some coaching from Denver's Toastmaster General, the Public Speaking badge came without a hitch.

Weekend hikes were no problem, but my parents and I had decided I should wait a year before going on an overnight. The last thing anyone needed was a reaction my first night out, and the year's wait would be a good break-in period before the test. It was around my thirteenth birthday that I enthusiastically told the patrol I'd be joining them the next time out, and they seemed pleased. They still didn't know why I'd bowed out of the earlier trips, although perhaps they "knew" and just hadn't said anything about "it."

I took charge of the food for our trip. We took enough chicken, potatoes, carrots, onions, bread, packs of raisins, chocolate bars, Life Savers, soup, powdered eggs, pancake mix, bacon, oranges, apples, and tins of deviled ham to feed the entire troop. When another Scout asked why we were eating so well, I just told him we were specializing in cooking and I happened to be the head chef.

That night was clear and cold, and as I lay down I felt the experience had been more than worth the year's wait. As I lay there with a feeling of confidence and exhilaration, I felt for the small leather pouch I kept by my side. In it were more rolls of Life Savers, sugar cubes, and a few trusty boxes of raisins. Throughout the expeditions and on all my excursions into the mountains with the Scouts or with the family, the pouch was my constant companion. If something went wrong, it was my life jacket.

Once in a great while, however, the life jacket failed and everything Scouting symbolized came tumbling down. On a particularly hot Saturday afternoon we took a hike through the prairie that spread east from the mountains. We had prepared to walk six or seven miles across some spectacular country. My family owned some land near the final destination, and I was anxious to share my knowledge of the area and its wildlife. I always wanted to show others how to walk quietly without scaring game, and while I myself never learned just how to do it, I made it a point to try.

We talked about the cactus, the grasses, the clumps of scrub oak and took breaks beneath an occasional cottonwood or pine tree. We watched for birds and gophers, marveled at the thin streams that disappeared beneath the hot sand and then reappeared a mile later surrounded by low willow. I had my pouch with me on my belt, but it was half-empty. We were only out for an afternoon, and since the territory felt like my own backyard, I assumed I could make it without any problem.

As the afternoon wore on, I began to feel the trip would never end. We kept walking and walking, and although the land was familiar it felt as though we were getting farther from reaching the end. I noticed that I seemed to be more tired than the others; and then, as always happens as a reaction progresses, my perceptions began to change. The plants became remarkably distinct. The sky became incredibly clear. As I gathered grasses to fill a collection book, I became obsessed with doing it exactly right no matter how much time it took or what anybody else said. The voices of the other Scouts seemed too loud, out of place, without sense or meaning.

Sweat began to sting my eyes. No matter how hard I tried I couldn't blot it out. Suddenly I didn't know where we were going. My eyes burned, but I wasn't sure whether it was tears or sweat. I kept trying not to break my stride, but was getting dizzy. "Get out of the sand," I said to myself, "you've got to get away from the soft sand and get onto solid ground. The body uses less energy walking over solid ground." But I didn't know which way to go. And the solid ground was covered with yucca and grass. I realized I couldn't hold together anymore and felt a rush of conflicting emotions flood through me all at once. I didn't want to cry, but I sobbed. I wanted help, but I didn't. My patrol leader came over, and soon the Scoutmaster joined him.

"My eyes, my eyes," I kept saying. They poured a canteen of water over my eyes. Still the sting continued. I couldn't see. Everything was bright spots and nothing would focus. The Scoutmaster put his arm around me and told me to take some candy. I took it. Other kids came around and he told them to leave. They did, and slowly I came to.

Somehow we made it the final few miles to his house. It was surrounded by beautiful ponderosa pine trees, and we sat at a table in their shade. Someone had put a glass of juice in my hand, and I could feel my body continuing its return. I kept looking at the bark of the pine tree. It was the same color as my neckerchief. The bark was beautiful, I said to myself, but beauty alone was useless. I caught fragments of conversation.

"We don't know," someone said. "It may have been his diabetes; it may have been just the sweat in his eyes. It may have been the heat." I felt again as if I wanted to cry. What if it hadn't been a reaction? What if I'd been weak and simply given in to something I should have taken in stride? And even if it was a reaction, why hadn't I recognized its signs? The Scoutmaster came over and sat down beside me. When he had put his arm around me in the field I'd felt relief. Now, even though he was as considerate as could be, his presence underlined my sense of failure. Worst of all, he was a friend of my father's and now knew both sides of my diabetes.

I loved Scouting and the adventures that were so important to my growing up. I'd joined the troop to prove I could do anything anybody else could, and had proved it all until that afternoon. While others told me not to worry, I felt I'd betrayed a trust with the troop and with myself, and wondered where to begin all over again.

13 · FOR THE RECORD

Testing my urine for sugar five times a day and keeping accurate records of my control were, I kept telling myself, reasonable medical expectations. It was only by looking at the tests that the doctor and I could develop a strategy for successful control. Somewhere along the line, however, I began to see the tests as an evaluation of personal success and failure as well as a medical record, and that's where the problems began.

I knew exactly the way the tests should look. The bright orange plus-4 tests should be avoided at all costs, and too many blue negative tests meant I was coming too close to reactions. The ideal chart would show a scattering of light green tests, indicating just a reassuring trace of sugar thrown in with the negatives. Unfortunately, my tests rarely came out that way. They were either blue or orange, and bounced from one to the other in a matter of hours. I hadn't felt the wild fluctuations during elementary school, but by the ninth grade they became daily occurrences. Carefully counting every single calorie and monitoring my every move might have brought them under control, but I had no intention of replacing my spur-of-the-moment living with a well-managed, moderate, and essentially boring life when I felt fine most of the time.

As I saw it, I had reasons to distrust the urine tests in the first place. My blood sugars changed so fast the urine sugars couldn't indicate where things really stood. Urine collected sugar only after it appeared in the blood, and by then the blood sugars might have changed. Sometimes the tests showed I was spilling sugar when I knew very well I was falling into a reaction. Besides that, some people's kidneys spilled sugar when it was present in only traces, whereas other people's kidneys could hold back a great deal of sugar before allowing it to spill over what was known as the renal threshold. The more I learned about urine tests, the less I trusted them.

I could also have explained my poor results by calling myself a "brittle" diabetic. Brittle diabetes meant the wild fluctuations were part and parcel of the disease. Fear was still another explanation. Negative tests looked great on paper, but at bedtime I'd often take an extra bowl of cereal just to make sure I wouldn't slip into a reaction during my sleep. Although it kept me safe throughout the night, the extra calories led to a high sugar the next morning.

When all was said and done, however, my perceptions felt like rationalizations. Poor tests indicated poor control, and made me feel I wasn't a very good diabetic. I wanted to hand in records that revealed a young diabetic in firm control of his disease. But the more I tested, the more impossible the goal seemed.

It didn't take long before my five daily tests dwindled to one or two a day and then down to two or three a week. Even when I did take them, I rarely bothered to record the erratic results. Instead of tests, I relied on gut instinct as an indicator, and most of the time it worked very well. The problem was that my doctor, who was a family friend and whom I respected a great deal, naturally expected a complete set of test results. Feeling compelled to take him something, I'd sometimes start up a flurry of testing a few weeks before the appointment. After a few days, however, my efforts usually petered out.

I felt caught in a bind. If I took in an empty record book, he, my parents, and even I would think I was an irresponsible diabetic who just didn't care, when that wasn't the case at all. If I told him I was doing fine without the tests, he'd quite rightly ask me how I could be so sure. So it seemed there was only one thing to do.

The night before an appointment, I'd put together the most realistic record book any diabetic has ever seen. A scattering of trace tests, a few empty boxes to show a few accidentally missed tests (nobody could be perfect all the time), a number of plus-4s (which proved it wasn't fake, because no diabetic would ever be proud of a plus-4 test), and hosts of plus-3s and negatives covered my bets. I took care to show the patterns that actually reflected the cycles of my diabetes. When I was out with the Scouts I showed a string of negatives; when I was sick there were plenty of highs. Knowing that nobody could keep a record book for three months without losing pencils and dropping it from time to time on a wet bathroom floor, I put in the appropriate smudges and water marks.

I knew very well that the grand deception wasn't right, and making up the charts gave me an odd feeling. In my "regular life" the truth meant a great deal. Lying to my parents, stealing from the till on my paper route, and cheating were all things I just wouldn't do. But when it came to diabetes, the rules changed as though my life and diabetes were two increasingly separate worlds.

For a good many years I thought I was the only diabetic who fooled around with his record book. Since then I've learned that that is not the case. In fact, when I've told the story of my record book, some diabetics would begin to laugh as they remembered the "adjustments" they made at one stage or another of their diabetes. Whether I would have done any better with the blood-sugar monitoring devices that are now available for home use I can't say for sure. They provide better accuracy, but are more complicated than a quick test. My hunch is that I might not have done much better with them than I did with my urine tests. Problems with a record book seem to be almost a common denominator in growing up with diabetes.

"You know," said Dick Evans, "the interesting thing is that you didn't take the most obvious route."

"What was that?" I asked.

"You could have said that the tests didn't reflect what was really happening, and that your internal monitoring worked just fine most of the time."

"That would have been unacceptable," I said. "They needed proof."

"I think that you, and perhaps many diabetics, keep record books for the wrong person. You felt beholden to the doctor instead of keeping the records for yourself. In some ways, the record book stimulated you to keep track of what was going on. But it wasn't all that important when compared with the records that you kept in your head."

"Those were the records I didn't fool around with," I said. "It was second nature to monitor myself like a hawk most all the time."

"But you had to learn how to gauge yourself from somewhere," said Dick. "Taking tests regularly in the early days, and checking yourself from time to time helped you learn how to interpret your sugars."

"I don't believe I ever saw it that way," I said. "I thought my internal radar system would be unacceptable to anybody but me, and only the written record would be valid in the doctor's eyes."

"From time to time he did need to see the tests," said Dick. "So the patterns you put down probably did help him. And I'm not trying to say that tests aren't a good idea. But in terms of your growth, you sold yourself short as a person. That is easy to do when the impression of what you think you're supposed to be is so strong. Records must be kept for the right person and in the right context. Understanding that is a challenge for all diabetics. Are they taking care of themselves? Or are they simply conforming to someone else's expectations? It's never all one or the other, but working through the difference between them is another part of growing up as a diabetic."

I suspect my doctor had tried to make it clear the record book was supposed to be no more than a tool, and I probably nodded my head in agreement without realizing how profound a point was being made.

"What would your response have been if he had said you don't need to be perfect?"

"I wouldn't have believed him and it would have annoyed me," I said. "Second-best isn't as good as best, and it would have felt like giving in or losing."

"Would you have liked for your doctor or your parents to have come out and challenged your records?"

"I'd like to say yes," I answered, "but it would have been tough. It's like I was going in two directions at once. It would have almost relieved me to have been confronted, but I was an expert at covering my tracks."

"Human beings," said Dick, "can be counted on to be ambivalent when it comes to talking about one's diabetes or other hidden and supposedly 'shameful' problems. But maybe one lesson we could learn from this is that doctors should go ahead and talk about things anyway. Somebody should be around to deal with juvenile diabetics even if they take the chance of being obnoxious as they make an opening for the diabetic to talk. And the diabetic needs to realize those tests aren't ends in and of themselves."

If I'd only seen that the tests and record books were tools and not commandments, it would have been so different. We could have talked about how 2s, 4s, and negatives felt and what steps might be taken to prevent problems. If the doctor had said, "How do you think you're doing today?" I might even have placed bets according to how I felt and then checked them with the test.

Unfortunately, that's not the way it worked. When my doctor looked through my record book for tests and patterns, he found them. He never asked if the tests were true, but neither did he compliment me on the fine work. Perhaps he knew all along and didn't want to upset me, just the way I didn't want to let him down. In any event, I felt a touch of relief and guilt when he closed the book and looked over to me.

"How's everything going?" he would ask patiently.

"Fine," I would answer, "just fine."

14 ◆ DAVE'S DIARY

Our family subscribed for years to the American Diabetes Association's *Forecast* magazine. It was written about, for, and sometimes by diabetics. Back in the '50s and early '60s it wasn't slick like *Time* or *Newsweek*, didn't have the heft of *Fortune* or the expertise of *Scientific American*. And unlike them, it couldn't be found at the local newsstand. It didn't even look like a conventional magazine. It was small, the home pictures looked like Brownie snapshots, and it lacked blazing headlines.

I would pick it up on lazy afternoons and thumb through it. There were recipes galore in most issues. Each had been field-tested by other diabetics and had the servings broken down into exchanges that would fit any diabetic's diet. The recipes avoided sugar, deep-fat frying, and excessive amounts of sour cream. *Forecast* recipes rarely found their way to our table. The idea of making an exclusively diabetic dinner for the whole family struck us all as impractical. My mother simply made special servings for me when we had complicated dishes. It became a regular thing to look over to the stove and see my small blue dishes standing beside the larger family casserole. I didn't mind the distinction in the least, and was glad the family didn't cater to my needs. The one meal we didn't know quite how to handle was my birthday. The watermelons planted with candles that we tried for a few years were truly mortifying, and as I remember we eventually ended up using angel-food cake and strawberries instead.

Forecast carried feature stories about diabetics taking vacations around the world on ocean liners and airplanes. The authors went into explicit detail about exactly how they handled the time zones, and how they counted out exchanges of Chinese rice or French onion soup. They shared the high points of the wonderful trips they managed to take in spite of their diabetes.

For the most part, their adventures weren't terribly exciting to a fourteen-year-old. I kept wondering what they saw and what they did once they got there. When I was an adult, I wanted to do more than cross time zones without having a reaction, more than just make it from one meal to the next without a reaction. Spending life simply managing diabetes wasn't very exciting.

Their stories were also suspect because for the most part they were about adults, with whom I couldn't and didn't want to identify. The only diabetes that really counted, it seemed to me, was juvenile diabetes. If older people had just not gained so much weight, if they had stayed healthy, they wouldn't be diabetic in the first place, I said to myself with adolescent certainty. Somehow their diabetes seemed like a character flaw. If someone really wanted to know about the disease, he should talk to a juvenile diabetic. My opinion didn't make much sense, was scientifically incorrect for the most part, and was horribly unfair, but I couldn't shake the feeling. The fact that juvenile diabetes was far more serious and its implications more foreboding gave me a feeling of pride. When someone said that juvenile and adult-onset diabetes might be two different diseases, I was thrilled. I didn't realize it then, but my prejudice was a common one, and for better or worse, there would eventually be the Juvenile Diabetes Foundation and the American Diabetes Association competing for the same dollars.

There were, however, two sections of *Forecast* that caught my undivided attention. The first was called "Young Folks Corner." Although it was only one very small corner of the magazine, it was expressly for kids. Kids between seven and fourteen wrote in telling how long they had been diabetic and how many units they were taking and concluded by asking for pen pals. Sometimes the pictures they sent in showed kids with big healthy smiles. Other snapshots showed rather lonely-looking kids who were desperately in need of a pen pal. Their letters were usually short, sometimes only two or three lines. Even after I'd passed the pen pal stage, I carefully read their letters and always wished they would go on longer.

Did they feel the way I did? Did they write their letters because they wanted to, or was it their parents' idea? Had they joined Scouts? Did they too feel different? I wouldn't ask diabetics questions about themselves in person, but print was a private message with a "time out" quality to it that caught my curiosity. Those kids knew something. We had the same disease. And I was curious to know what made them tick.

The best place to learn how diabetics ran their lives, however, was in "Dave's Diary." Dave was a diabetic who related his adventures near the last page of each issue. Although he was an adult, he had grown up with diabetes, so both juvenile and adult-onset diabetics could identify with him. During the years I read *Forecast*, Dave found a girlfriend, married her, became a father, and like most of the television fathers of the 1950s held a steady but unspecified job. Most of his life was an open book, and I looked to him for all the guidance I could find.

Dave handled his diabetes very well. If my memory serves me correctly, he once reported he and his bride-to-be were out dancing when he suddenly realized he hadn't eaten enough dinner to make it through the dance. He didn't hesitate to ask her if they couldn't take a break. She thought that would be fine. They sat down, and the steady and reliable Dave asked for a small glass of juice. Once recharged, he invited her back to the dance floor. As I remember it, they became engaged shortly thereafter.

Another time Dave attended a dinner party and found that foods were served which diabetics shouldn't have. Using all his discretion, he ate only tidbits of the difficult foods and tried to balance his meal as best he could with available staples. After dinner he politely excused himself and walked around the block several times to burn off the excess. Then he returned to finish the evening. Nobody took note of his absence. There were no problems. He handled it perfectly.

Still another time Dave woke up one morning with a fever. He naturally tested, recorded a plus-4 test in his reliable record book, and immediately called his doctor, who was pleased to get the call despite the time of day. Dave followed his instructions to a T and had recovered by the next issue.

Dave's wife was a model of understanding. When she became pregnant Dave wrote about all the preparations they were making, and when the baby was born (it wasn't diabetic), he announced to all the readers of his diary that he had become the complete family man. Personally, I was glad we could get away from his family life and back to his diabetes. As a young teen-ager who had decided never to get married no matter what, I more or less resented her intrusion into his life. Still, she was sympathetic, supportive, and a good cook, could tell instantly when he was slipping into a reaction, and was now a winning mother.

There was very little about Dave that wasn't picture-perfect. Whatever the challenge, Dave could handle it. His questions had answers. A single Life Saver could pull him out of a reaction; a brisk walk around the block could restore his sugar to normal. When he had the slightest question about his treatment, a quick call to his doctor solved it. Basically, he never got caught.

But I sure did. Compared with Dave, I got caught all the time, and I began to wonder how anybody could be as perfect and well balanced as Dave. He never hit panic buttons, never sneaked a Milky Way bar or got caught tasting honey just to see what it tasted like. His perfection both attracted and bothered me. He was telling a true story, I presumed, and there must have been a real Dave somewhere, but was he telling the whole story?

What did his wife do when the meals were accidentally late? Didn't she get upset when they missed connections? Didn't his doctor have too many patients to get a call from Dave when his urine sugars showed a plus-4? I liked and respected my doctor, but the thought of calling him at seven in the morning every time I spilled sugar was ridiculous.

In some ways, I looked up to Dave. In other ways, I didn't want to be anything like him. My diabetes wasn't like his. Mine changed wildly. His moved gingerly, carefully, when it moved at all. The answers that worked for him just didn't work for me, and while I doubted if I'd ever have the even-tempered maturity of a Dave, I wasn't sure I wanted it.

I knew why the travel stories, the "Young Folks Corner" and "Dave's Diary" were in *Forecast*. The travel stories were there to provide assurance to diabetics afraid of travel. Dave provided a textbook example of how diabetics can make it through life and work with their doctors. "Young Folks Corner" gave kids a chance to reach out and realize they weren't the only diabetics in the world.

All those messages were important. But it was the unspoken stories behind the examples that captured my imagination. Who was Dave? And who were those kids who, for reasons I can't really explain, I felt I couldn't write but wanted to know? I read *Forecast*'s every issue, and put it down wondering what it was really all about, who those people were, and who I would one day be.

15 • CAUSES, CRUSADES, AND DREAMS

One afternoon Martin Luther King, Jr., passed through Denver, and my mother and I went to hear him speak. He was late arriving, and we waited for him in a large, jam-packed downtown church with a sense that it would be a meaningful and memorable experience.

Beside us sat a blind woman with her guide dog. It was a golden retriever. We quietly talked with her for a few moments, and then I reached down to pat the dog. She heard the faint jingle of its tags as I brushed its harness.

"I'm sorry to ask you this," she said, "but are you patting the dog?"

"Yes," I replied.

"Please don't," she said, almost apologetically but with firmness. "I know you don't mean any harm, but if I ever lose the complete affection of this dog, I lose my eyes as well."

"I'm sorry," I said drawing back, "I didn't mean—"

"I know you didn't," she said gently; "no one ever does." She said her words so simply, so truthfully that I never forgot them. The normal way of doing things wasn't always the right way of doing things. Good intentions could get in the way.

When Dr. King came in, the sanctuary fell silent and we all turned to the pulpit. He had only a few minutes to be with us, and apologized that he couldn't spend more time. The headlines were ablaze with the civil rights movement in the South, and in some ways Denver seemed a long distance away from Mississippi. But the issues were the same. It felt like a gathering of friends who understood the changes of heart that needed to occur. Dr. King may have been in a hurry, but he didn't seem rushed. He asked for a moment of prayer as he concluded, and then moved on his way. The blind woman left with her dog, and we all filtered out of the church.

Causes, crusades, and dreams became an increasingly important part of my life. Sometimes I understood why, and sometimes I didn't. Don't be so dogmatic, my mother kept saying. She was right, but I wouldn't slow down to consider my opinions or to take a good look at myself. I wanted to set things right and to be the first one to make great discoveries. My intensity came from an insistence that all things could change for the better, and diabetes was no exception.

Each year at Christmas the creativity of our family and a fling with magical thinking came together. My mother was the instigator, and we followed her lead. Back in California, she had hit upon the idea of producing an opera with marionettes. It sounded farfetched, but with her drive and determination anything was possible. She had us handcrafting the marionette heads from papier-mâché, making hands of tape and wire, and carving their joints from wood. Strings ran from each to a complicated double-cross control stick that we held in our hands. Once dressed, the marionettes (she insisted that we never call them puppets) took on their own personalities and turned Mother's daydream into a reality. They could sit, stand, bow, and fall. They could be amusing or dignified. When Mother wasn't watching, we had them high-jumping and levitating from the stage with incredible ease.

Menotti's *Amahl and the Night Visitors* was the chosen work. It was in English instead of Italian, it told a Christmas story, and its theme was healing. My mother and I were attracted to it almost as though it had been written for us. She and I, who so deeply shared my diabetes, shared the opera's secret hope as well. It was almost as though if magical thinking hadn't existed we would have found a way to create it through our Christmas production.

We had seen the opera in Los Angeles, listened to the album regularly, and knew it practically by heart. Before my voice changed I even daydreamed about being accidentally discovered as the next Amahl. What I didn't have in my voice could be made up for with sincerity and an understanding of what the opera was all about. It never happened, of course, but the dream was very real. I wanted my story to be Amahl's story, and believed they could be the same.

Amahl wasn't diabetic, but he was a crippled boy with a bright imagination. He lived with his mother, who both struggled to make ends meet and worried about his tendency to tell tall tales. One night after he'd told her about an unusually bright star that seemed to have a tail, there came three knocks at the door. It was the Three Kings, who asked if they could stay for the night. Once she overcame her disbelief she agreed, and they walked in bearing gifts and gold for the Christ Child.

During the night she tried to steal some of their gold for Amahl and was caught. When the Kings eventually told her whom the gold was for, the full meaning of the star and their voyage became clear. For a moment they shared a sense of wonder and purpose. As the Kings prepared to leave, the crippled Amahl suddenly understood what his gift to the child might be.

"But Mother," he said, struck with inspiration, "let me send him my crutch. Who knows—he may need one."

"But that you can't, you can't," she gasped. Not believing her, and with his mind on the gift, he held out his crutch and took a single small step without it. They were watching a miracle as he took a second, and then a third. The newly born Amahl began to dance, to fall, to laugh, to run with the grace of a young man discovering there were no bounds. Each time I heard the song I made the story mine, wanting to believe that its message was true. He gave his crutch, and in the giving became cured.

We invited the entire neighborhood to see the show several days before Christmas, and each show was like an opening night on Broadway. We worried about dropping the marionettes, wondered if our whispers could be heard, made sure the dog was out, and fought the jitters as my father turned down the house lights.

It was a family event in every sense of the word. Three-year-old Doug opened the corduroy curtains. My mother manipulated

89

Amahl, who had a special thread to drop his crutch at the magic moment. I had Melchior, the wisest king. My brother Jack, two years younger, took Balthazar, and Ken, five years younger, took Caspar. It was understood that Jack and I would keep a sharp eye on Ken throughout the performance; if we didn't, our kings might be standing on stage while Caspar snoozed through a trio. Once in a while someone would ask if Caspar hadn't had a bit too much to drink before show time. But he was a little deaf anyway, so it really didn't matter if he missed an occasional cue by a second or two.

The presentation became a high point of our neighborhood's Christmas. It was our family at its best, at its warmest, at its most creative. Its connections with diabetes ran deep for all of us. We asked the neighbors, after the show, to send in contributions to the American Diabetes Association. As for me, I wanted to be Amahl. Whatever he gave I wanted to give. If he could be cured through sheer desire and goodwill toward men, perhaps the same could be true for me. It was a story of healing and hope, of dreams that made their own truth. It was a story of magical thinking. And we threw ourselves into it with all the love and hope of Christmas.

16 · ECHO

Feet presented an unusual challenge. Although my feet looked and probably felt like the feet of almost any other high school sophomore, book after book emphasized that a diabetic's feet needed specialized attention. Each day they were to receive a gentle bath in warm (not hot) water. They were then to be carefully dried with soft towels, inspected for any sores, and treated with creams and lotions. Diabetics were never supposed to go barefoot. If our nails were thick, they should be clipped by somebody else. We were supposed to make extra sure our shoes fitted well, that our feet didn't get overly sweaty, and that our socks were very clean.

Needless to say, the instructions seemed abnormal and sissy. The thought of gently bathing my feet after taking a shower was just too much to swallow. And nobody needed to tell me to buy shoes that fitted. When my feet were wet, they dried themselves off somewhere between the bathroom and my bedroom, leaving trails of water up and down the hallway. Thick nails or not, I'd be on my deathbed before I'd ever let anybody else come and clip them for me.

In my sophomore year, however, the nitpicking messages about foot care and the chance of infection in diabetic feet struck home. As so often happens, what appeared to be a small mishap that wouldn't affect anyone else magnified and moved quickly into the danger zone for me.

As a diabetic, I was not immune to colds. I caught them just the way everybody else did, no more and no fewer. Illness, however, threw my diabetes out of control and sent my blood sugars sky-high. Even when I became nauseated and lost a meal, I'd have to take some extra insulin. It felt strange to take more insulin when I was eating less, but my doctor explained that my body was working overtime to conquer the infection and needed all the insulin it could get. When I lost more than one meal after taking my shot, slow sips of defizzed and tepid Coke could keep me on the safe side of things.

One fall afternoon in the midst of tennis tryouts, I suddenly felt dizzy and upset to my stomach. Knowing it wasn't a reaction, I went home, threw up, and lay down. There was no chance of keeping down any snack or dinner, so we brought out the Coke. It wouldn't stay down either. By nine that evening everything was out except the bitter digestive juices, and they too kept coming up. By midnight, I finally fell into an exhausted sleep.

To my surprise, everything felt fine the next morning. I took a standard shot, went upstairs to breakfast, and ate without any problems. Because of the siege the night before, we decided I should stay home for at least one day to recuperate.

The morning passed calmly, and by lunchtime I wished I'd gone to school. I had long since determined I would not be a sickly person and disliked giving in to myself by missing a day. By two o'clock, however, I began to feel woozy. By three I had to keep flat on my back, and by five the vomiting had started again and wouldn't stop. We brought out the Coke, and once again it wouldn't stay down.

The next morning I took my shot thinking the storm had passed, but that afternoon it hit with the same vengeance. Meanwhile, my diabetes was falling apart at the seams. My sugars were on a roller coaster, always adjusting to whatever had just happened and unable to find an anchor. The doctor told me to increase the dosage and take it easy on meals even when I felt fine. The plan made sense, but left me famished each noon. One day I ate a dish of cold macaroni and cheese. It tasted out of this world, but it didn't last beyond three o'clock.

That morning I stubbed my left little toe against a doorframe. Like most stubbed toes, it hurt like hell. After dancing around for a moment or two, I looked down and spotted a small trace of blood just where the cracked nail met the skin. I squeezed it to get rid of the pain, and watched the drop of blood ooze from beneath the crack.

Although it would be risky, a quick rip across the top of my nail would remove the remaining tab without doing further damage. I tightly squeezed the toe and then quickly pulled the cracked nail. To my horror, it ripped down to the root instead of across the top, and the bleeding began in earnest. I could have kicked myself for not letting well enough alone as I sat there holding it and blotting up the blood. Magical thinking entered the picture as I decided to simply ignore it. Nature will take its course and heal if you just don't think about it, I said to myself. Over the next few days, I kept the nail hidden beneath my sock, hoping the wound would go away. When I finally looked at it, the tiny piece of remaining nail was surrounded by red skin. It began to itch, and the redness began to spread. Meanwhile, the nausea returned each afternoon right on schedule.

Losing the battle on both fronts, we called the doctor. I was feeling scared and desperate, doubting that I had the strength to make it through another siege. He came immediately out to the house and examined me. He saw my foot, and asked how it happened. I told him I'd stubbed it so hard the nail had been torn off naturally. He said it was infected, that we needed to get to the hospital that very afternoon, and that I had a flu called Echo.

Practically delirious, I pleaded for something to drink. My mother handed me a wet washcloth to quench the same kind of thirst I'd had in Maine seven years before. For the second time, I lay in the back seat of a car as we drove to the hospital. Everything was out of control. My mother kept telling me to suck on the washcloth, that everything was going to be all right. I didn't know whether she believed it or not. She seemed frantic to get me there.

I don't remember going into the hospital, but do remember waking up with an IV in my arm. The hospital staff monitored my blood sugars regularly, and had outsmarted the nausea by avoiding my digestive track entirely. My strength slowly returned, and within a few days the redness in my foot faded. I didn't know exactly what gangrene looked like, but became convinced they were helping me fight it.

After four days they slipped out the IV needle, and I began to eat the vegetarian meals served by the hospital. My roommate, who took great pleasure in frustrating the Adventist nurses by ordering blood-rare steaks as often as possible, admired my courage as a diabetic and wondered if he would be able to follow all the rules and regulations. I didn't tell him about the foot rules I'd neglected. And to tell the truth, I still don't carefully bathe my feet the way the books admonish. But the next time articles appeared about foot care in *Forecast*, I knew at first hand what they were talking about. Whether it sounded sissy or not, diabetic feet were vulnerable and diabetes could be a precarious disease.

17 ♦ FAMILY

"When I was a little kid," said my younger brother Ken, looking back on our growing up together, "I remember going into the bathroom and playing with your equipment. I was almost envious of it, and playing with it made me feel special too. Your being diabetic was something extra you got to do that we didn't get to do."

"Me too," said Jack. "I was dying to get my hands on that syringe. And to this date I've never done it. I just wanted to get an orange and jab it."

So that was how my younger brothers felt about my diabetes. When we were together as kids, I hadn't known. Talking about diabetes was like bringing up a touchy subject, so we tried not to bring it up much. It wasn't until we had all left home and started our own families that we were able to look back and share our reactions. As it turned out, I was the diabetic but we had shared diabetes.

I have three brothers. Jack, the one two years younger than I, was a quiet and confident athlete. Ken, who manipulated Caspar in the marionette shows, had an incurable sweet tooth and was the baby of the family until Doug came along. There is a thirteen-year spread between Doug and me. For him, diabetes hadn't changed anything because in his eyes I was never a nondiabetic.

"I don't remember the orange thing at all," said Ken, laughing at Jack's coveting the diabetic orange, "but I do remember Mom telling me to test myself every once in a while just to make sure I wasn't diabetic, and that really scared me."

"It was dangerous to be too thirsty around our house," teased Jack.

"I mean we didn't have a chance on a hot summer's day because somebody would jump up and want to test us. I'm exaggerating, of course, but the thought was there."

"I loved going to friends' houses," said Ken. "They got Kool-Aid and cookies when they came home from school. We never had anything like that at our house. That may be one reason why I didn't bring kids to my house that often. It could be. I never thought about that until now." With a sweet tooth like Ken's, a diabetic brother could really mess things up.

"He's right, you know," said Jack, continuing his tease. "Other kids' houses definitely had more sweets. There is no doubt about it. They had those deviled marshmallow cookies and stuff. All we ever had was fruit."

"Did you resent me for that?" I asked.

"Sure," said Jack, trying to get serious, "but it wasn't really a resentment. It was just a fact of life."

Just as I'd accepted a positive, no-problem approach to diabetes, so had they. Being positive was almost a requirement for membership in our family. My mother once studied music with a Denver conductor who had the habit of asking a question and then saying, "Say yes" before it could even be answered. Ours was a Say Yes family, even though diabetes wasn't always a Say Yes proposition.

"I don't believe we minimized what was going on," said my father. "We all knew diabetes was a life of sickness. But I do think we bent over backwards to try and make it as normal as we could."

"Normal," said Ken, "but hushed. I was told never to talk about it."

"I don't remember telling you that," said my father with surprise.

"Nor do I," added my mother.

"Oh, yes," said Ken, "the impression was very clear. Larry's diabetes was something we shouldn't tell our friends about. Never. It was absolutely a private family affair."

"We were open about the camp," said my father. "We may have told you how to handle it at school, but I didn't think it was covered up."

"I had the same impression as Ken," said Jack. "It wasn't completely taboo, but it wasn't the kind of thing you went around and talked about."

Sometimes it is hard to understand what is passed on in a family. The messages that get through aren't always the ones intended. Hopes, values, and fears all find their way into the lives and imaginations of kids independently of a parent's words and intentions. Kids pick up the denial, the magical thinking, and the source of most emotions with an uncanny ability and then reflect what they find in their own lives. As they do, they hit their parents' emotional buttons and begin to test limits they weren't even supposed to know about. Family strategies have a way of backfiring. Parents pledge to raise their kids differently from the way they were raised, and frequently end up realizing they haven't changed a thing.

In our case, we fought hard to make sure diabetes never became a reason to do less. We skied, camped, fished, took vacations, did our chores, sang in the choir, got into fights, and made sure diabetes didn't get in the way. In so doing, we pushed our doubts and curiosities underground, where they surfaced differently for each of us.

"I thought it was special to have a brother who was diabetic," said my youngest brother, Doug. "I can remember being down at the grade school and telling a few of my friends my brother was diabetic. That made me sort of special, because I knew what it was and could tell them about Larry's shots. I had no idea what diabetes really was, but I did know it was a disease."

"Were you ever embarrassed about it?" asked my mother.

"No. It was special. Friends of mine would come home and say, 'Is he the one? Is he the diabetic?' It was like a big mystery."

"As parents," said my mother, who was hearing these stories for the first time herself, "we were never told how to prepare the siblings. I don't even remember thinking about preparing you, except in emergencies with insulin reactions."

"In the back of my mind," Doug said to me, "I've always kept a little fear of your reactions, especially when it comes to the car. I remember once when you had one driving down the New Jersey Turnpike with Mom and me. It was terrifying. You were driving and she had to suddenly grab on to the wheel. Then we had to pull into a parking lot, and I remember you eating a Hershey bar.

"It's been a long time since you've had a serious reaction, but even now when I'm alone with you in the car the thought is there way in the back of my head. I think, Okay, you could have a reaction, and

97

then what if? What if you had a reaction and went out of control?"

"I knew what to do if Larry had a reaction," said Jack, "but they still scared me to death. There was always a fight. Mom yelling, 'Take this' and Larry screaming, 'No, I don't want it, I don't need it!' They were embarrassing, too. I was always afraid of Mom saying to me, 'Jack, go to somebody right now and get some sugar!' And I'd have to go to a stranger and ask. It would have sounded so dumb. I never had to do it, but I was afraid I might have to bail you out."

"But there is another side to reactions," said my father. "Very early in the game someone told me that no one ever died from a reaction. You can be out cold on the floor, you can have a convulsion, but it is not terminal. To me, that was always a very comforting thing. And there were steps we could take. When we gave you the syrup, you came back like magic."

Karo corn syrup was our home remedy for bad reactions. It was so thick I couldn't choke on it, and so sweet it would pull me back almost instantly. We kept a jar of it in a kitchen cupboard, and the one ugly bottle lasted for years and years.

"I have no recollection of your ever becoming mellow," said Doug. "All I remember is the terror of the time."

"Same here," said Ken.

"Going into a reaction," I said, "gave me the feeling of being painted into a corner. I tried so hard to avoid problems that when one came along it made me lash out. Some of the anger was the chemistry of the reaction itself. But I've always wondered how much was simply fighting to get out of being diabetic in the first place."

"Larry," said my father, "I'm surprised at your emphasis on never being caught or making a mistake. I'm not aware of that as something we tried to transmit to you as parents."

"Well," said my mother, "I think we were scared to death that something might go wrong. And a mistake would mean terrible problems."

"Was my diabetes more on your shoulders than on Dad's?" I asked, wondering if that accounted for their differing views.

"I was around more," she said, "and a lot of our family life, especially meals, revolved around me."

"Either way," said Ken, "reactions always upset the family balance."

"That's why I hated them," said Jack. "It had very little to do with Larry. Mostly they upset Mom and Dad. To tell you the truth, that's why I didn't like reactions."

"In all honesty," said my mother, "I would have to tell you I cannot say I dealt with your reactions with equanimity. And even though the doctor said they weren't fatal, to see you unconscious was frightening."

Diabetes was not something we could avoid. It was something we both openly shared and kept secret. It had influenced my brothers' lunch boxes, led to the creation of a camp for diabetics, and certainly upset the family balance.

"I think for me," said Jack, "and maybe for all of us, it was a peripheral thing in our lives. I had my own things to do, and Larry's diabetes was simply a fact."

"What?" I asked, wondering if I'd heard him right.

"There was no point in talking about something that would make you feel bad," said Ken. "I thought it was wiser to have you think I didn't even notice it."

"I thought," continued Jack, "that our family had a very normalized atmosphere. There was no kind of pity leveled on Larry. He was not a special person—he was just like the rest of us."

Right there was the paradox of diabetes in our lives. A few moments before, they had spoken of fears that never left their minds and about the family balance that reactions could unexpectedly threaten. Now they were telling me it hadn't been much of an issue at all. We had all bought the bill of goods that says diabetics can lead "normal" lives, and ended up concentrating on the word "normal." Diabetes was like an invisible envelope around each of us that had kept us from being as close as we seemed and as close as we wanted to be.

How does a family learn to accept diabetes? The same way a diabetic does. It is a long process of trial and error, of learning what can and cannot be changed, what can and cannot be believed. There is no easy way to do it. In many ways, our positive approach worked very well. But as we finished our talk that night, I couldn't help wishing we'd tried it twenty years before.

18 · COMPETITION

Senior year I wanted to prove myself. How much of that was the result of being diabetic and how much was simply the result of being seventeen years old is an interesting question that didn't go through my mind much at the time. As I saw it, the rules were simple: high school was competition, and I wanted to compete.

The year began when Mike Koch stepped off the bus in Denver on a bright September morning. He was an American Field Service exchange student from Geneva, Switzerland, and we had been selected as his host family. Mike spoke fluent English, immediately called my parents Mom and Dad, and blended right in with our family. He and I shared a room, and we spent hours talking about world politics and comparing European with American skiing. As with most brothers, there was some competition mixed in with our friendship.

I told Mike about my diabetes right off the bat, and with his quick mind he seemed to understand very well. He was a superior student, and could analyze an argument instantly. He could also catch the contradictions that seemed to characterize my ideals. I threw myself into the political campaigns head over heels, asking everyone I knew to both push for integration and vote for Goldwater at the same time. My arguments with Mike over politics were constant, provoking his European sophistication and my American emotionalism all the way.

Athletics, however, brought home our major competition. Mike was a champion runner, one of Switzerland's best. When he went out for cross-country, he promptly set a school record that lasted for several years. I had won a small skiing cup once, had competed in some good tennis tournaments, but deep down didn't consider myself an athlete. After all, Mike wore our high school's bright yellow letter sweater, not me.

Looking to prove myself, I found English class. Although I never learned to spell, detested grammar with a passion, and resisted the discipline of workbooks, I had an imagination for literature as vivid as that of my teacher, Mr. Armstrong. Walking into Room 110 was like walking into England itself. One of his daydreams involved putting a map of London on the back wall. He didn't have an ordinary map in mind. He meant a map ten feet long and six feet high that would further transform our room into the capital city of the sceptered isle.

The idea caught my fancy and suited my qualities. It was clearly something nobody else would do. It required patience and persistence and allowed me to run the show however I saw fit. It also gave me a chance to make a lasting mark. So while Mike trained after school for cross-country, I spent afternoons creating the biggest map of London the world has ever seen. As word of my project spread through the school, teams of other kids began to check in for duty at two thirty. When it was framed with mahogany planks in the early spring, *The Denver Post* came to take a picture of what was by then known as "Pray's Map of London."

Looking at my name on the stupendous map struck me as somewhat embarrassing—but to be honest, I could have told Mr. Armstrong to leave my name off it and didn't. Mike and I now both had our names engraved on a school wall. But famous as the map was, there was a big difference between the physical glory of athletics and a map of London. High school athletics had long evoked images of locker rooms for the privileged, and I had generally kept my distance from locker-room talk and varsity competition. The problem was that maps and tennis simply weren't the same as football, basketball, or track. I knew it wouldn't be right to leave high school without overcoming my fear. Like it or not, I had to join Mike and go out for track.

My whole stomach tightened up as I walked into the first team meeting, and I was relieved that nobody seemed to notice me. Workouts would begin the next day, said the coach with a tough tone and knowing locker-room kind of laugh. The whole team groaned and laughed as though they knew exactly what to expect.

When the bell rang the next day, I ran to the concession stand, bought the sweetest-looking candy bar I could find, and promptly ate it, hoping to avoid any reactions during the afternoon's torture. When the athletic-looking crowd headed for the locker room, I casually drifted along with them. They changed clothes, and I changed clothes. They went out to the gym, and so did I. They were as relaxed as could be, and I faked it as best I could.

We spent all afternoon running up and down steps and across the gym floor until our legs were ready to drop off. But the farther we went, the better I felt. I kept up, didn't complain, didn't have a reaction, and most of all discovered I didn't need the freedom that came with an individual sport to make it as a diabetic. At the end of practice I was on Cloud Nine, even enjoying the locker-room talk as everyone relived each moment of the afternoon's agony.

A week later the weather warmed and it was time to make the big move from flats to spikes. Mike had bought a new pair, and carried them with him as the coach lined us up for announcements. I was greatly impressed with Mike's spikes. It seemed they had been magically honed for Olympic competition. I hadn't bought any myself, figuring you had to be on the varsity team and have some kind of secret card before earning the right to go in and buy an official pair of track spikes.

"How many of you jokers don't have spikes?" asked the coach. Actually he didn't ask, he snapped. About ten of us raised our hands.

"Well," he said gruffly, "over there in that box we've got some extras for those of you who haven't managed to get your own yet. Go ahead and use them for today."

My spirits soared. This was really serious track! We stepped out across the floor toward the cardboard box. After about ten yards the coach saw me moving with the rest of the kids.

"Pray," he said, "you won't be needing them." My heart fell to the floor. He couldn't mean it, but he did. I looked over at him, but he had turned away and was talking with an athlete. It was a moment of total humiliation and anger. I vowed somehow, someday, to prove him wrong. If I ever coached I would give spikes to everybody, crush the elitism of high school athletics, and never forget what a track team might mean to the hopes and dreams of every kid.

I eventually chose the mile as my main event, and soon realized I wasn't a born runner. No matter how hard I tried, others would pass me by after the first lap. In fact, I never even went to a single meet. I was persistent, ran my assigned laps religiously, but failed to reduce my times. Mike, who was the team's star, had the good grace not to talk much about its victories.

Going out for track, however, was a victory in my growing up as a person and as a diabetic. The last day of the season the coach came up and spoke directly with me for the first time.

"You're in shape now," he said. "Good season."

"Thanks," I said. I felt that I should be resentful, but I wasn't. What he said was true. I felt strong and fit. My self-doubts had been partially vanquished, whether or not anyone else noticed. Diabetes hadn't been a problem and my courage hadn't failed. Fifteen years later, when the track team I built and coached won the New England Championship for the third straight year, the vows and lessons of my 1965 track season came home in a new way.

Shortly after the end of school Mike prepared to go back to Geneva, and I made plans to leave home for a summer job in Maine. When I lay down in bed the night before our departures, I knew that all future returns would really be visits. The thought carried with it both a sense of eager adventure and a feeling of sadness tinged with remorse. I fell asleep thinking of all the trips we'd taken as a family, of the marionette shows, of ski weekends, of Scouts, of weeds and gardens, of all the times we had done things without letting diabetes get in the way.

In the middle of the night I unexpectedly woke up and found myself sobbing. I kept thinking of my parents and was sure I had caused too many problems without giving sufficient thanks. My diabetes had been a burden, and I wanted to apologize for the tensions everyone had borne so well. I wanted to go back and do it all over again, making it so much better that diabetes itself wouldn't be there. My tears came with the recognition that it was too late to give overdue thanks, that it was too late to change things. After a while the emotion passed and I fell back to sleep.

The next morning I took my shot as usual, went to the family breakfast at seven o'clock, and left home.

19 ✦ DAVIS JUNCTION

It took me a while to learn how to laugh at myself as a diabetic. Taking good care of myself meant always anticipating what I'd do if the unexpected threw my plans off track. Simply making sure I'd make it to meals sometimes turned ordinary events into a comic opera. Boarding the train in Denver for the trip to college, I double-checked the rolls of Life Savers in my pocket (in case meals weren't served on time), made sure my insulin was in the bag (knowing there wasn't a pharmacy on the train), and felt for my wallet to confirm for one last time that I had some money to bail me out of any emergencies (like derailments) on my way to Beloit College in Wisconsin via Davis Junction, Illinois.

I stayed up most of the night in the Vistadome watching the isolated Nebraska ranches pass us by as we made our way through the star-filled night. It was an exhilarating feeling to be heading into a world where no one knew me, but I wanted to be sure I'd make it through the night. From time to time I tested myself just to make sure I wasn't close to a reaction, and kept taking small snacks to carry me over to morning.

When we crossed the Mississippi River the next morning I asked the conductor about Davis Junction. He said there wasn't much to it, adding that not many people got off there.

"Is it a full station?" I asked, wondering if there'd be a café in case I needed a meal.

"Not really," he said. I made my way to the dining car and ate a huge breakfast wondering why I'd never heard of Davis Junction. When the conductor called out the stop, I noticed that none of the other passengers made the slightest move toward their bags. On both sides of the train were stands of trees and fields of corn, but there was no town in sight. We kept slowing down and finally came to a stop in what seemed to be the middle of nowhere. The conductor pulled down the steel steps, and I climbed down onto a small red brick platform in front of a field of corn. For a split second I wondered if the whole episode wasn't some kind of practical joke, and imagined hiking through the fields to a farmer's house where I'd beg food and explain the intricacies of diabetes.

There were, however, three others who were in the same predicament. We all stood there waiting for the last car to pass and then gazed upon a dilapidated freight depot and a few farm buildings.

"Is this Davis Junction?" I asked, just to make sure.

"I guess so," said one of the other students. We were all reassured when fifteen minutes later a car from Beloit pulled up to meet us. By then it was about two o'clock, which meant I had to begin planning dinner.

Now, I presumed that the college would have some kind of dining facilities. But to tell the truth, I had myself half-convinced that perhaps college students were so busy with their studies they rarely stopped to eat. It was plausible that the dining halls had been phased out in the interest of academic excellence. I didn't dare ask anyone in the car because it would have sounded like a dumb question. Either they'd say, "Of course not!" and I'd appear unsophisticated, or they'd say, "Sure there are dining halls" and wonder why I'd asked.

When we arrived at the college, a dorm resident showed me to my new room. He told me my roommate hadn't arrived yet and then asked if everything was okay.

"Yes," I said, "but I do have one question. Where is the nearest restaurant?" I didn't ask him if the college had a dining hall.

"Just around the corner there is a little pizza place," he said.

"How do I get there?"

"Go out the door, cross the campus, and you'll run right into it."

"Thanks." He left, and my thanks wasn't very convincing. Walk-

106

ing across campus, I wondered how on earth I'd survive eating pizza for a year. Once I got there I was glad the place had hamburgers as well. I ordered one, figuring it would hold me for the rest of the afternoon.

About six I heard some people talking about dinner as they were walking out of a building. Sure enough, it was the dining hall. What a relief. People really didn't get so lost (or so I thought at the time) that they avoided the basic necessities of life. I went in, selected an acceptable diabetic meal, and sat down as though I were home. It was all going to work out.

That night I had to tell my roommate about my diabetes. I had no idea how to approach the subject, and would have avoided saying anything if I could have, but if I did have a reaction that night he would need to know what to do. One always needed to be prepared.

"Could I talk to you for a second?" I asked after he'd unpacked.

"Sure," he said. He was an Easterner from Cape Cod, Massachusetts, and had put a bottle of Canoë men's cologne on his shelf. I thought it was perfume. Nobody from out West worth his salt would ever use something like that, I said to myself.

"There is something I need to tell you about. Don't worry about it, but you should know just in case there are some problems."

He looked up with a quizzical expression.

"I'm diabetic," I said, deciding to just plunge right in, "and I have been for eleven years. So if you ever see me acting rather strange, it is because I am in a reaction. Most people think you should never give sugar to diabetics, but that isn't true. So if you see me being kind of crazy, belligerent, dizzy, pale, or just not being the normal person I usually am, I need some sugar. A Coke would be fine, or some juice if you can find it."

"Okay," he said. It didn't strike me until later that he had no idea what "normal" meant when it came to me.

"One more thing," I said. "If I say I'm all right I'm probably not, so don't hesitate to just kind of force the sugar down."

"If you say so," he said, probably wondering if he still had time to change roommates.

"Thanks," I said, glad the ordeal was over and hoping there wouldn't be any problems.

Life settled down after the first few days, and the routines of college life and a sense of self-discipline made my control fairly easy. I learned to study long hours, and attacked my work full force. Book passages were underlined, notes carefully typed; research papers had more quotes than I knew what to do with. Convinced everyone else was smarter than I was, I relied on methodical persistence, and was thrilled when I didn't flunk out that first term. I went home for Christmas with a fairly sophisticated vocabulary, although nobody else seemed to take notice.

As the newness of college wore off, however, my attitude toward diabetes began to change. Perhaps it was the cynicism that seems to come with college; perhaps it was just my outgrowing some old approaches and learning to relax; but for whatever reason, I began to feel that diabetes was in fact a liability. And I began to resent it. The denial of many years caught up with me, and I began to search for a total solution.

The drift had commonplace beginnings. I wanted, for example, to sleep in on Sunday mornings once in a while instead of getting up and going downtown for a diabetic breakfast. After all, my body couldn't tell the difference between a Sunday and a Monday morning and everyday was supposed to be the same. Nevertheless, I began to sleep in and found that while it messed up my control, I did it anyway. I'd take extra units to burn off meals that were too large, and exercised whenever I felt like it instead of setting up a regular routine. I joined a fraternity thinking that ready access to a kitchen would help me take better care of myself, but the plan backfired as I began to maneuver around the balanced meals I needed. In fact, snacks sometimes replaced meals entirely. By the end of my first year and a half of college, I had little desire to walk the straight and narrow and a great desire to find an escape.

20 ◆ PASSPORTS

In the winter of 1967, a group from Beloit was scheduled to attend the University of Rennes, France, and live with French families. I had taken French since the eighth grade, and Mike and I had hoped for a return exchange. Part of the reason for attending Beloit in the first place was the chance to study abroad, so I applied for the program and was accepted despite the diabetes.

Europe marked a major transition for all of us. I didn't know how I'd handle my control, but hoped the year's slide would end. For my parents, Europe marked another stage of letting go. They came with me to New York for the departure. Whereas my mother was filled with excitement and concern the night I left, my father's emotion came out as confidence in whatever I might do. He was the one who delighted in and supported these adventures, and knew they had to happen whether or not anyone was ready.

As we ate dinner I tried desperately to remember what the world travelers had said in their *Forecast* articles. How had they handled the time zones? Did they eat meals or just take a host of snacks until they safely arrived? Should I just forget time zones and take my shot with the dawn in Iceland? That idea was rather romantic, but it might not work. I could have kicked myself for never carefully reading the experiences of other diabetics who had crossed the sea.

I gave my parents a last hug; checked my insulin, roll of Life Savers, and passport; and then walked through the New York drizzle to the plane. To my surprise, the stewardesses brought out a meal soon after our departure. Not quite sure just what to do, I gazed at it for a moment calculating calories and time zones.

"The idea," said the fat man next to me, "is to drink as much wine and eat as much food as you can and then go to sleep." It sounded like a marvelous idea, but it would never work for me. I picked at bits and pieces of the dinner; took a few modest sips of wine, figuring it was time to get ready for France; and sat back checking my passport for the fifteenth time. The thought of being detained in a Luxembourg jail as a diabetic without a passport did not please me in the least.

We landed in Iceland with the morning light, and I decided to take my shot and roll with the punches. As long as I was spilling sugar (and I was), everything would be all right. Several meals later we landed in Luxembourg, where it pleasantly surprised me that the world still looked flat. I knew Iceland wouldn't be a problem because it was "up" on all the maps. But Europe was simply "across," and one secretly never knew what might happen over there on the edge of the earth.

When we arrived in Rennes, France, the next afternoon, my new family met me at the station. Both Monsieur and Madame Beltan were doctors. It didn't occur to me until months later that I was assigned to them because of the diabetes. It wouldn't have made a difference had I realized it, however. The new language, a new culture, and a family that accepted and enhanced my spirit all made for a change of pace that overcame my resentment of diabetes. There were no reactions, no close calls. When I found they ate dinner at eight instead of six, I simply took my morning shot two hours later and everything worked out just fine.

New beginnings, however, don't last forever, and the three months in France soon came to an end. Having studied for five straight terms, I felt it was time for a vacation, and while I was looking forward to joining Mike in Geneva, I wasn't quite sure what to do with the free time I'd have on my hands. There is a strong connection between diabetes and one's sense of direction. When I took a positive attitude toward myself, my control improved. When uncertainty got the better of me, control went down the tubes and my resentment toward diabetes surfaced.

On the outside, my activities in Switzerland were as outgoing and varied as ever. Mike and I skied down glaciers together in the Alps, ran through the countryside to keep in shape, and took courses together at the University of Geneva. My French continued to improve, and life with his family was a joy. Had anyone asked how everything was going, it would have looked fine. But on the inside I wasn't sure where I was headed, and magical thinking was about to launch its first serious crusade.

Mike and I planned to take a week-long trip through southern France. Whereas I'd meticulously arranged my provisions for most of my trips, this time I decided to do exactly the opposite. For once in my life I wanted to give impulse a chance and not play it safe. I threw my insulin and syringe into the glove compartment the same way I'd toss a shovel into the back of a pickup. On this trip there were no rolls of Life Savers, no testing equipment. I took a minimal amount of money. A distinctly clear thought ran through my mind as we set off for France. Take your shots, it said, but don't do anything else. You don't need to hit panic buttons when events don't conform to the needs of diabetes. Ignore the whole thing, and you'll be all right.

It was a breathtaking trip. Country roads lined with shade-giving trees, rivers that sprang from the sides of mountains, streets aglow with the warm southern sunlight, and the cool palaces at Avignon were all alive with history and imagination. But my experiment with magical thinking wasn't working. Reactions came like a string of exploding firecrackers, each one worse than the last. Once it happened in a restaurant as we waited for a meal. Twice it happened late in the afternoon as we drove the car. I'd fall asleep and Mike couldn't wake me up. He had to rush and find some sweet syrup and then pour it down my throat. I would come to; wonder where we were, what had happened; and then reassure him it had been just a slight slip that wouldn't happen again. But it would.

As I look back, it is amazing I didn't come to the logical conclusion that ignoring diabetes wouldn't work. Magical thinking, however, isn't a matter of logic. In fact, it's like a cat that has nine lives. Instead of going away forever once it didn't work, it came back with increased momentum. Instead of eating more to protect myself after the reactions, I ate less. Meals on the road were expensive, I said to myself, and I didn't want to spend all that money just to be well fed.

If the French had rolls and coffee for breakfast, I would do the same. I had no intention of asking for eggs and bacon when Mike and I ate breakfasts in village squares filled with sunlight as pleasing as Impressionist paintings. I would defy common sense. The very thought of "successfully managing diabetes" by following the rules made me want to break them all the more.

"You must have felt pretty angry toward yourself and your disease," said Dick after I'd told him the story.

"I just didn't want to take care of myself on that trip," I said.

"Did you consider that dangerous?"

"No. In fact, it was exciting wondering what was going to happen. I wasn't trying to do myself harm, I just didn't want to bother for once. When I took the shots it was slam-bang and then I tossed the equipment back into the glove compartment. I don't think I even used cotton swabs."

"Did you ever think that if you didn't take your insulin at all your diabetes would disappear?" Dick asked, wondering how far my magical thinking might go.

"No," I said. "I didn't even consider that. I knew if I went without insulin I'd get sick in a hurry. I took it because I had to, and then tried to forget about it. But I've since learned that there are diabetics who do refuse to take their shots. They usually end up in a hospital, which seems scary to me. But that is the way they apply magical thinking, and to my surprise, it's not that uncommon."

"The one thing about not eating," said Dick, "is that you would eventually come out of it. Did you perceive that your approach was safer than if you ate too much or didn't take your shot?"

"I hated the feeling of spilling sugar," I said, "whereas getting close to a reaction was like playing a game of Chicken with myself."

"I think it is important to recognize magical thinking and how it shows up in diabetics," said Dick. "We all have an inborn tendency to try to control external reality by controlling our interpretation of it. As we grow up, we develop increasingly elaborate ways of deluding ourselves by manipulating our perceptions of reality.

"Look at the athlete who believes that if he works hard enough his team will definitely win. Then if his team doesn't seem to be winning, he'll feel the spell is broken and tend to give up. Eventually he'll hopefully learn how to continue playing hard even though he knows he's going to lose. That is a prerequisite for a winning team. I think it is the same learning process you had to go through with your diabetes.

"But diabetes isn't a winning proposition. It demands a lot of care and has a lot of complications that get worse with time. A diabetic can look at that and give up, or try to ignore it through a desperate kind of magical thinking. When that happens, things can really gang up on you. That's what happened on your trip."

Mike and I returned to Geneva several days early, and a week later I met up with an American friend who was passing through with some companions on his way to Italy. Despite the reactions, I wanted to continue the experiment with freedom as I traveled with them.

"Larry," said Mrs. Koch at my departure, "I can't believe you're going with so little."

"This is all I need," I said, picking up a small satchel and shoulder pack.

"Okay, if you say so," she said with affection and concern in her voice. She knew I was headed for trouble and could sense something wild and irrational in the whole scheme. But what could she say? And what could I say? I told them I'd return before I left for the States, gave them all a big and thankful hug, and jumped aboard a train bound for Italy.

21 ⋄ LIMITS

Magical thinking was a matter of limits, and there were two more tests to be taken. Both were risky, and both took me to the brink. As I write about these experiences it is almost hard to believe that they actually happened. I never thought of myself as a gambler or as a person "out of control" of his life. The thought that emotions might be more powerful than reason seems to open the door for all kinds of problems, rationalizations, and excuses that were the opposite of the way I wanted to be. But like it or not, there is no getting around the fact that in the summer of 1967 I was hell-bent on wanting to get rid of diabetes and followed my magical rebellions to the end.

We bought tickets for an overnight train bound from Rome to Venice. A curious urban beauty filled the station that evening as we waited for the train. The thick afternoon light gave a kind of glow to the tracks and people who walked up and down the platforms speaking a host of different languages. My friends had Eurail passes, which meant they traveled first class. I bought the cheapest ticket available and took a seat in the second-class section. They felt bad I couldn't sit with them, but I told them not to worry, that we would meet up when we arrived in Venice the next morning.

I felt unusually tired as I sat down and stared through the window. A pushcart vendor walked alongside the train selling snacks.

"*Gelati*," he hollered. "Ice cream, ice cream." Hands reached through the windows passing change and grabbing the bars. I had had only some fruit and bread for dinner, and knowing it wouldn't be enough, I bought an ice cream bar to hold me through the night.

An Italian family with four kids asked if they could sit with me, and I responded in French that it would be fine. They had a large picnic basket with them and asked me if I'd like to join them. Not wanting to inconvenience them or to say yes because I was diabetic, I politely declined. When they finished, they leaned back in the seats and began to go to sleep. Outside, it was dark, and the train's steady rhythm quickly make me drowsy. I checked my satchel beneath my feet, looked up at the small packsack to make sure it was still there, and fell fast asleep.

Exactly what happened between my falling asleep and my waking up in the Bologna infirmary surrounded by police I'll never know, but it had to be a mixture of both miracle and disaster. I had heard about diabetics who had been picked up as drunks or addicts when in fact they were only in a reaction. They would be thrown into jail, laughed at when they pleaded diabetes as the reason for their outlandish actions, and left to suffer until someone realized what was going on. To be in need and have nobody realize it was a frightening thought. Throughout high school I'd worn a Medic Alert bracelet just to make sure I wouldn't be caught. Fortunately, I'd never needed to use it. In Europe, however, I didn't have the bracelet with me.

When I woke up, all I knew was that I must have been through a reaction. I was lying on an infirmary table. Above me was a fluorescent light, and beside me were police and a woman who wore a bright green dress.

"Où sommes nous?" I asked in French. A policeman produced my passport.

"Lawrence M. Pray," he said with a slight smile, "American."

"C'est moi," I said sharply in French. I couldn't tell if I'd been rescued or arrested.

"You American?"

"Oui," I said, bound and determined not to speak English. Somehow speaking English would seem like an admission of defeat. Larry Pray the diabetic spoke English.

"Where are my things?" I asked in French.

"This is all you had," said the policeman, holding up my small satchel.

"No packsack?" I asked. He didn't understand the word, so I pantomimed. He shook his head. My insulin, I thought; I've lost my insulin and all my money. I began to explain that I was diabetic, that I needed to both eat and find a pharmacy. They listened carefully, and when I showed the nurse my syringe and kept saying "Diabetic" she seemed to understand. All of a sudden it hit me how kind they were trying to be, and how sharp my responses had been. Without them who knows what might have happened?

"Where did you find me?" I asked.

"*They* found you," said the nurse, pointing to the police.

"Where?"

"Beside the tracks."

I'd like to write that the experience scared me. But it didn't. In fact, I felt a sense of exhilaration as I climbed aboard the next train to meet up with my friends in Venice. It was a bright day, and despite the fact that I'd lost almost everything I felt I had nothing to fear.

When I returned to the States two weeks later, my family met me at the Denver airport. It was good to see them again, but returning home also felt like returning to the challenges I hadn't been able to escape. They asked about the reaction in Italy, and I told them the whole story. Mom said I looked tired and thin, and while I wanted to refute her, she was right.

My mother, Ken, and Doug had planned a trip to Ghost Ranch in Abiquiu, New Mexico. She was scheduled to take a course in choral conducting and asked if I didn't want to go along. In the "Say Yes" tradition, we thought it would give me a chance to recover from the string of reactions and for us to spend some time together as a family.

The ranch itself was beautiful. Wide-open plains surrounded it, and a few sentinel-like monuments stood above the whole view. While she attended classes, I tried to get involved in activities around the ranch and thought about the hopes I'd held for my European adventures. I couldn't help thinking about the diabetes I'd hoped to escape, and disliked the idea that I was now supposed to give in and take care of myself like a normal diabetic. Cynicism, anger, and resentment all replaced the enthusiasm that had buoyed me before through difficult times. Looking in the mirror, I didn't like what I saw.

In an effort to break my mood, I went one morning with a ranch crew to fix some fences. We jumped into the truck, drove up a can-

116

yon, and spent the morning setting some new fence posts. A reaction began to move through me, and its growing presence made me increasingly angry. I threw myself into the work all the more, trying to ignore it and make it go away. Fortunately, we stopped work and headed back to the ranch for lunch before I got into serious trouble.

That afternoon I took a walk across the desert alone. If there was any way on earth, I told myself, that I could take this disease and simply leave it there in the sand, I would do it. The thought wasn't a daydream. It was a clear, calm, and distinct thought. If I believed with all my heart and soul that diabetes could be left there in the desert, when I returned from that walk it would be gone. At that moment, magical thinking was no longer a stage of my life. It was an all-or-nothing proposition. Ghost Ranch, I thought. The name was an exact fit. I too felt like a ghost.

I walked back and joined the others at dinner. Fighting a desire to fast, I ate a small meal, chatted with some friends, and turned in feeling spent by an impossible dream and an inescapable reality.

That night the bottom dropped out. Convulsions from a reaction threw me out of my bunk. I turned blue, choked on my tongue, and fought off everyone who tried to help. I had gone into the desert with everything I had, and diabetes had hit back with all its frightening power.

"That whole week had a strange feeling to it," said my brother Doug. He was six at the time, and had slept in the bunk beside me. "I remember waking up and it was just pandemonium. Of all the times you've had reactions, I thought that was the closest you came to dying. You had superhuman strength when you had a reaction, and it took all of us to hold you down."

"You were purple," said my mother. "You were being asphyxiated, and I knew you were dying. You had convulsed yourself onto the floor from the bed and were making awful sounds. I was in the next room when I heard you.

"I just couldn't hold you down, and went banging on all those doors at the ranch. Ken was running around for sugar, and I was trying to get help and hold your mouth open while a man squeezed the juice from an orange down your mouth. Another man was running to the Coke machine."

Finally the juice began to work, the violence left, and life began to return. My brothers looked at me with expressions of fear and concern. The men who had held me down slowly left for their rooms. My mother was crying. I didn't know just what had happened, but felt I'd been on the edge of not coming back. None of us knew where to turn, what to say.

"Did you know, Larry," said my mother as we talked about it. "that this reaction happened on August fifth, your birthday?" I'd forgotten that. For a long time after Ghost Ranch, however, I dreaded the month of August. August was always the end of something, whereas September was a crisp beginning.

I still find it hard to think back on Ghost Ranch, and I hope I never see days like those again. Denial and magical thinking had taken me to the brink of death, and left me just this side of it. I saw clearly that my life could not continue with diabetes as an enemy to be escaped. I now knew for the first time with inner certainty that it really would never go away. There would be no more experiments, no more brinksmanship. I left those dreams at Ghost Ranch. The road to acceptance entered a new stage.

22 ✦ PANDORA'S BOX

"What you went through," said Dick as we talked one evening about Ghost Ranch and its lessons, "is a universal experience. It didn't look like it at the time, but it helped you come to terms with yourself."

I suppose it's always true that growth is more easily said than done, more easily conceived than understood. The lessons of Ghost Ranch seemed almost embarrassingly simple in hindsight. I was diabetic, and there was no getting around it. Some things you can change; others must be let alone. After a Herculean battle, I had begun to learn the difference.

In some ways, it was a foolish battle. Ponce de León's search for the fountain of youth had always struck me as an amusing tale until I finally realized I had embarked on just as magical a journey. Pizarro's quest for El Dorado was irrational too—just as irrational as the hope we all harbor that somehow old age and death may pass us by. They won't, of course, and there was no fountain of youth or El Dorado. But that is the kind of lesson we all must learn as we mature. Being diabetic simply meant I had to learn it sooner. When I walked too far out on a limb, diabetes snapped right back and hit with full force.

"Other people use other things to try and learn that lesson," said Dick. "We eventually find out, much to our dismay, that our bodies are very limiting compared with our minds and imaginations. We try to prove that our bodies won't limit us. Taking drugs, alcohol, driving cars fast, jumping out of airplanes, hang gliding, skiing down

Everest—those are all attempts to prove that 'It ain't so,' that we aren't really mortal and that we can be heroes. Sometimes it takes a long time to understand that we are mortal. In your case, diabetes accelerated the lesson."

"Diabetes didn't give me an out," I said. "It forced me to come to terms with myself one way or another."

"That's right," said Dick, "and it isn't like cigarette smoking, where something might happen to you in fifty years. Diabetes makes it an immediate thing. If you don't take a shot, you'll spill sugar and go all to pieces. If you don't eat, you'll have a reaction practically on the spot. Your getting to the end of magical thinking was like completing an initiation stage in your development as a person."

As we talked, it struck me that growing up with diabetes was like the story of Pandora's Box. It was one of those stories I'd learned in elementary school that had always stayed with me. The young Pandora was a beautiful girl who lived in a world without fear, war, famine, or poverty. Disease didn't exist. In her home was a box which she was told to never open. At first she didn't even consider opening it. But then curiosity overcame her, and although she knew better she lifted the heavy lid for a glance inside. As soon as she did, a host of evil spirits flew out far beyond her reach and disease infected the world.

Pandora was simply human. She knew from the best authorities available exactly what she was supposed to do. But like most of us, she couldn't resist finding out what would happen if . . . For her, disease and evil spirits came from the same source. She saw disease as a scourge, and all these years later, so do we. No wonder we try to deny diabetes in the first place.

As she sat weeping and frightened, there came from within that dark chamber a small voice asking to be let out. With great courage, considering what she'd already seen, she opened the lid again and the spirit of hope entered the world. Although the evils couldn't be forever conquered, they could be endured as long as there was hope.

With magical thinking, I had taken the soft voice of hope and turned it into a storm. I had to learn that hope is a virtue, but pretending is dangerous. Diabetes taught me the difference. It was a hard lesson to learn, because who could have imagined that hope could be a hindrance? The best part of life was trying to make dreams come true. When Amahl walked, the audience was moved. When the blind and deaf Helen Keller touched water and said the word, we saw limitations left behind and her spirit ignite. When my friend *Paddle-to-the-Sea* finally reached the sea, when we saw the first pictures of Earth over a pale moon, when "in spite of the difficulties and frustrations of the moment" Martin Luther King still had a dream, life itself took a quantum leap.

As one diabetic said to me, "I always felt I had to fix myself. And fixing myself really meant that I couldn't be diabetic. Or it meant I had to be the 'perfect' diabetic, which was impossible." He could have spoken for me. We both had to learn the difference between fantasy and hope, just the way Pandora had to find out what was in that box and then reconcile it with the world she had once had and couldn't have again.

"There may have been some other things going on back then too," said Dick, "and they could have made a real difference." He mentioned that some new studies are revealing how moods can influence diabetes. I had long known that when I felt great I needed less insulin. When times were depressing, my diabetes became uncertain, my body stalled, and my insulin requirement went up.

Moods can be a tricky business, though. They both cause problems and forewarn of reactions. I remember once laughing at an ordinary joke when I noticed everyone else had long since stopped laughing. I really did think the joke was amusing, but reached for a Life Saver just the same. When I get depressed, I tend to get sleepy. The same thing happens when I'm spilling too much sugar. In either case, it may take going out for a run or some other dramatic change of pace to get myself back on track. If activity doesn't do the trick, then I can settle in for a good night's sleep.

According to Dick, one psychiatrist had studied the insulin requirements of diabetics undergoing treatment for depression. The doctor discovered that as the depression subsided, the insulin requirement was almost cut in half.

"Back when you were a teen-ager," said Dick, "you were probably going up and down a lot emotionally. Most adolescents are very sensitive. They get depressed about some little thing that a younger

121

child or an adult wouldn't get upset about, and then bounce back higher than a kite the next day. That could have been a major factor in your control. Adolescence can be a slippery time for diabetics."

"I could feel that instinctively, but never read about it back then," I said.

"Well," said Dick, "I think it is an old thing that is just now being widely noticed and studied."

There is much about diabetes that is just now being observed. New techniques that weren't even a glint in the eye when I was a young diabetic are now making a major difference. Some diabetics control themselves by taking as many as four or more shots a day. They are able to monitor their sugars with electronic machines and have achieved far better control than was possible with my one shot of NPH a day. Those techniques could have evened out my control a good deal, but might or might not have led to acceptance. Techniques alone don't teach Pandora's lesson. The best approach in the world must eventually be understood from the heart and then applied as a reflection of both personal growth and medical care.

I had never heard of the serenity prayer at the time, but I wish I had. Diabetes had helped me take some first small steps toward wisdom. "God grant me the courage to change the things I can," went the prayer, "the serenity to accept the things I cannot change, and the wisdom to know the difference." The Ghost Ranch incident didn't lead to an automatic acceptance. Far from it. But it did end one stage and lead me into another.

"Acceptance," I said to Dick, "sure was a longer journey than I ever thought it would be."

"Be careful," he said. "When you talk as though acceptance is ever complete you tend to lose it. Thinking about a completed acceptance is part of the problem, not part of the solution."

Acceptance is one of the mirage-like words. Just as one never quite finishes growing up, one never fully accepts diabetes. Along the way, however, there is much to be learned. Denial and magical thinking were the first stages. Willpower would be the next. Pandora's Box had been opened, and I'd learned it couldn't be closed. Now its elusive forces had to be contained.

23 ♦ PICKING UP THE PIECES

A doctor recommended spending four days in a Denver hospital when we returned from Ghost Ranch. The stay would allow for regular monitoring of my blood sugars and provide a pure environment for charting and then calming my wild fluctuations. He had taken his residency at the Joslin Clinic in Boston, Massachusetts. I didn't know much about Joslin, but had heard it was a kind of Mecca for diabetes research and care. Patients from all over the world went there to get regulated and to learn about their disease. He was a stickler on the need for absolute control.

With patience I awaited his prognosis, and predicted in advance what he was going to say.

"Larry," he would say, "we've got to get you regulated."

"I know."

"Do you understand how diet, exercise, and insulin all work together?"

"Yes."

"And do you realize that the better your control the less chance there might be of future complications?"

"Yes."

"As long as you understand how all the pieces fit together, you'll be able to stay right on top of it. Your control is up to you."

That was what he would say, and that is the gist of what he said. All the medical and moral evidence supported his understanding. I'd known for many years what should be done to treat diabetes, and now needed to get down to business. It was as simple as that. At issue was my character. After all, there were doctors, hospitals, research centers, nurses, and insulin itself all charting a path toward diabetic control, and there I was like a recalcitrant child being taken to task for something he'd known about for thirteen years. A strong person could control diabetes, and a weak person let diabetes control him. Accepting diabetes meant conquering it.

Willpower. Uncomfortable resignation. Anger. Those were the elements of the third stage of my journey through diabetes. Willpower because that was the only way to control the disease, and who could argue against the wisdom of being the "perfect" diabetic? Resignation because, unfortunately, there was no escape from facts that needed to be faced. And anger because despite all outward appearances, I felt cornered by a disease.

"This picture you had of the perfect diabetic is something that I'm sure most diabetics share," said Dick Evans. "But in terms of your growth, it is not a picture that should be taken too literally. It's as though the doctor needed to say, 'Here are the perfect results we want. But it is not essential that you give us those exact results. We'd like a reasonable approximation of them. You've got to find the limits of your diabetes without really hurting yourself.' It's the same kind of issue you faced with your record book. The diabetic must realize that he or she is the boss, not the doctor."

"If my doctor had said that back then," I said, "I doubt I would have accepted it."

"Why not?"

"I'd known for a long time I was in the driver's seat. So I would have said, 'What kind of games are you playing with me? Everybody knows that best is better than approximations.' And besides, I'd seen diabetics who cheated all the time and they ended up in serious trouble."

"But the nature of human beings," said Dick, "is to deal in mixed messages. And there is no such thing as perfection in anything human beings do. The attempt to achieve perfection is an attempt in life that has been amply described in literature as one which is punished by the gods. Diabetics are no exception to that. When you feel compelled to go against that and to achieve this elusive ideal that seemed so much better than you, anger and resignation can't help entering the picture, especially when you fight it. I suppose you toyed around with this stage years earlier with your record book, but now it entered the rest of your life as well."

It was to take me seven years to work through the willpower stage. They were seven paradoxical years. My life took on directions I found exciting and deeply rewarding in both personal and professional ways. When my attention turned from my life to my diabetes, however, I had a long way to go.

When the doctor in the Denver hospital outlined what we were going to do, he didn't ask about the magical journeys, and I certainly didn't think to tell him. The complicated blend of life and disease didn't count for much beside the serious business of diabetic control. It didn't strike me until years later how odd that omission was. We both knew I'd come within an ace of losing my life, yet neither of us even approached the question "Why?"

"The first time I ever heard of magical thinking," I said to Dick, "was the night you told me about it. For most of my life, the whole approach toward diabetes was future-oriented."

"What do you mean?" asked Dick.

"Treatment was built around moving toward an ideal. I spent most of my time, and I think the doctor did too, comparing me with the 'perfect' diabetic and then wondering how we were going to get there."

"Why didn't you bring up the rebellions?"

"I didn't even consider it. We were both so determined to get things straightened out that the idea of stages of growth might have confused things."

"I bet that's a problem most diabetics have with their doctors. Approaching it that way is a protection for both of you. As long as you and the doctor talk about tests or diets, it's safe. As soon as you start talking about personal experience, it gets fuzzy for all of us pretty fast."

"Well," I said, "conforming to his goal was the name of the game, even though it didn't work. It's easy to see why a disease like diabetes can so easily become tinged with rebellion and guilt."

"It may be very important," said Dick, "that patients go over their failures with their doctors. What you learn from your mistakes is critical, both for your own growth and for your control as well."

"I keep thinking that part of the bind," I said to Dick, "is that we keep trying to assume we shouldn't have any problems in the first place. We'd like to think we're too sophisticated to be swept off our feet by a fling with magical thinking."

"That's what we'd like to think," said Dick, "but that isn't the way human beings are built."

"I don't think I could have eventually come to an acceptance without going through some of these epic struggles."

"They should be expected," said Dick. "Acceptance isn't instantly achieved, and people don't grow up according to 'the rules.' The struggles are part of the process. We should keep in mind that compliance is one thing, and growing up as a unique individual is quite another."

As I lay in the Denver hospital, I felt like a guinea pig that had come in for retraining. The hospital staff took five or six blood sugars a day, brought in my meals regularly, and took my temperature even though I wasn't sick. It concerned me that the tests would reflect the sugars of a static world instead of my normal life, but the doctor told me not to worry.

Before long he felt it was time to try a new kind of insulin. Insulins, he explained, came in a variety of types, each of which had its own timetable. Whereas NPH peaked about nine hours after injection, the quick-acting regular peaked in only two or three hours. Semilente did the same thing as regular, but then stretched its maximum action over a four-hour period. Lente insulin peaked from eight to sixteen hours after injection. The strongest-acting of all was Ultralente, which didn't wear off for more than thirty-six hours. By mixing the various types one could avoid the peaks and valleys that came with NPH alone. He suggested a mixture of Lente and Semilente, which seemed fine by me. In fact, there was enough magical thinking hanging around to make the switch seem like leaving a beat-up Ford for a limited-edition Maserati. Then came the kicker.

"To make this work," said the doctor without missing a beat, "you'll have to take two shots a day."

"What?" I said as though I hadn't really heard him.

"One in the morning and the other at nine in the evening. Two shots will really help."

I reacted like a wounded pincushion. One shot a day hadn't posed much of a problem, but two shots a day was like packing somebody else's quota of shots into my life! I wondered if the damage could be sustained. Almost every diabetic book had charts showing exactly where shots should be taken on a rotating basis. The outside of the thighs, the hips, upper arms, and abdomen were the major target areas. If sites weren't rotated, the tissue could eventually lose its ability to absorb insulin. Still worse, it could eventually atrophy.

Wanting to avoid problems, I had always taken care to rotate my sites. I had somewhat skinny arms and not much fat on my sides, so I generally used my legs. They had enough room to last a lifetime as long as I was taking one shot a day. But two shots meant twice the damage, and I quickly imagined black-and-blue splotches on both my tissue-deadened legs.

And there was a second consideration. Nine o'clock was a strange time to take a shot. Before dinner would have been convenient, and before bed even better. But nine o'clock would be smack-dab in the middle of everything. Even Dave of "Dave's Diary" hadn't had to excuse himself from life for a nine-o'clock shot!

These impressions, of course, made absolutely no difference. Nor should they have. If the doctor said two shots a day, it would be two shots a day whether I liked it or not. My body would just have to absorb the blow. The next morning a nurse brought in my first injection of Lente and Semilente, and I waited all day for a surge of sustained energy and control. Needless to say, it didn't come. Even the nine-o'clock dose couldn't usher in a new age of diabetic control all on its own.

I didn't realize then that my whimsical hope that a new insulin would solve the problems was a perception commonly held by many diabetics. New equipment and technology can be almost like a new Christmas toy. Fascination with them gives the appearance of acceptance and a willingness to achieve control when it may be no more than a passing phase motivated by the hope that through new methods the problems of diabetes can be overcome. New dosages,

127

new insulins, and new techniques can significantly improve control. But there's no magic, and hope eventually settles down into the realization that so far there are no cures.

Two days later, I left the hospital and returned home. Although it was fall, I was officially on leave from Beloit. I signed up for some courses at the local junior college, but for the most part that fall was a kind of diabetic sanctuary. It was a time to make sure one day led to the next without incidents, and that is precisely what happened. I became resigned, in a sullen, practical sort of way, to my disease.

A month after my release from the hospital, I went back to the doctor's office for an appointment. I had eaten a somewhat makeshift lunch, and knew in advance my sugar would be higher than it should be. It was. When he saw my reading he was concerned, and I couldn't help feeling discouraged. A predictable picture of just the way things should be ran through his mind. The same picture ran through mine.

"Come on, Larry," I said to myself. "You could do it better if you'd just try a bit more. What's the problem, anyway?"

That question went through my mind all fall long. The sanctuary hadn't provided an answer, and by December I could hardly wait to get back to college. There the competition would pit me against others instead of myself.

24 • EXERCISES

The logo of the Joslin Diabetes Foundation used to show a chariot driver confidently reining in three powerful horses. One was diet, one insulin, the other exercise. The majestic driver had mastered them all. No one horse was dominant. All three worked as a team at the will of their master.

In the extensive guidebook given out to patients in 1978, there were some eighty pages of information. Explanations of calories, exchanges, insulin, foot care, sick-day rules, and blood sugars took up nearly all of those pages. Exercise received a mere one page that listed the number of calories burned by such activities as trotting a horse, playing squash, washing dishes, or driving a car.

I do not mean in any way to belittle the Joslin Clinic. It has been a tremendous diabetes resource for me. When its new unit was built, a fine exercise room was included for patients who wanted to use it. But despite the central role exercise plays in the life and imagination of a diabetic, there isn't much said about how to harness its powers.

Of the three horses, exercise was the one I liked best. I knew exactly what it would do and could limit the extent of its action. Whereas insulin worked according to its own schedule and food was a necessity to keep up with the insulin, exercise had fewer built-in requirements. When I wanted to run, I ran. It could restore a high blood sugar to normal or move me toward a reaction. The uplifting

129

ease that came after any extensive workout could transform a bad day into a new beginning. To me, exercise was the best way to compensate for an error. And that was the mistake.

Like most people, I assumed staying in shape ensured health. If I had to be a diabetic, I would at least be a strong diabetic. The stronger the better. It wasn't too great a step from that notion to its not-so-true companion: through exercise and willpower diabetes can be contained. Sports, which were a great way to take out one's aggression, became a way to try to conquer diabetes. What had taken one page in the guide became 80 percent of my care.

Other diabetics, I observed years later, had some of the same problems giving exercise its proper place as I had. One mother had a diabetic son who didn't take good care of himself most of the time but exercised with abnormal vengeance. Another diabetic exercised so much that his doctor finally told him to tone down, and still another remembered sports as the only really solid part of his high school education. For all of us, it seemed as though exercise was the most available horse in both a practical and a magical sense.

Such single-minded devotion, however, had its problems. Exercise was supposed to be a joint partner in the triad. Like meals, it should have been regularly scheduled. After all, if one of the three horses simply kept the other two in line and never had a chance to establish its own rhythm the team couldn't work as designed. For me, the consequences caught up with me in a strange way.

One day my tennis coach walked through the locker room as I showered after a workout.

"You've really gained weight," he said.

"No, I haven't," I shot back. "I'm in shape."

"Ten pounds," he said with a smile as he left. I went over to the scale and weighed in at an astounding 178 pounds, a good fifteen pounds over my usual weight. Evidently the makeup meals after runs had brought in too many calories. All the exercise could do was bring down my sugars.

I knew, of course, that I couldn't up and fast for a week to cut my weight, but that is exactly what I wanted to do. I needed desperately to follow a routine and put exercise in its proper place. But the intensity of my efforts kept going into short-term tactics rather than

130

long-term strategies. If I was high, I wanted to get low. When too low, I bailed myself out with whatever food was available. On both sides were extremes. It felt as though I were fighting on three fronts with only two hands. The more I strove on any two, the more the third popped up and caused problems.

A lot of effort went into those midmorning and sometimes even midnight runs, and a lot of rebellion surfaced in an inconsistent diet. A lot of anger went into the forceful containment of diabetes. Overall, it didn't work, and my frustrations began to surface.

For a short while there was another diabetic in our fraternity. I still don't know where he came from and didn't know his name, but I did know he had great difficulty with his diabetes. He didn't stay in shape, and when he got into trouble he seemed to give in.

One summer night there was a party going on in our building, and the booze was flowing rather freely. Part of being diabetic meant avoiding alcohol and drugs, and for the most part I went along with the guidelines. Both would interfere with my blood sugars, and could so easily confuse my system that I couldn't tell which way I was headed. Most people enjoyed the sensations of losing control. I was just the opposite. On that particular night, however, I had a hankering to find out what would happen if I had too much to drink. Needless to say, there were plenty of people who wanted to help me find out. I ate an ample dinner to tide me through any storm, and began to drink. Many glasses of wine and shots of vodka later, I had a hankering to get into a fight.

Now, I would like to say that I was so beside myself I didn't know what I was doing. And it would be nice to say that an evenly matched bare-fisted brawl ensued. But that was hardly the case. I knew exactly whom I wanted to hit. I got up, announced my intentions, and headed toward the other diabetic's room. Once I found him, I lunged at him before my shocked friends (who hadn't believed I was serious) could pull me back. The unsuspecting diabetic was so startled he scarcely knew what was happening. My friends hauled me back to my room and declared the party at an end. The rest of the night made me decide I didn't want to get drunk again for a long, long time. When I woke up, there was no question as to whom I'd really hit that night, and it certainly wasn't the other kid. He reminded me of

131

everything I was afraid I might become and might already be. In short, he caught my projected fears.

"That," I said to Dick, "is one of those stories I can laugh at now, but I didn't tell it much a few years ago."

"It's a problem most of us have at one stage or another," he said. "It's based on a revulsion, on things we're afraid of in ourselves. For you, it happened to be your diabetes."

"That's a dangerous feeling to have," I said.

"Dangerous, but common. It's like the censor who tries to get rid of things he doesn't like."

"When I started drinking," I said, "I was kind of saying that diabetes could be damned, if you know what I mean."

"I know exactly what you mean," said Dick, "and that's probably why you hit him. A lot of anger was building up in you about diabetes. He just happened to be in the wrong place at the wrong time."

Part of the problem in seeing diabetes as an enemy to be controlled through willpower was that its relationship with "the rest of my life" wasn't explored. As long as I saw diabetes as a parasite, I didn't see what could be learned from it along the way. The challenges I faced academically, for example, were much the same as those I faced in coming to terms with my disease. As usual, the link showed up unexpectedly.

I had signed up for a course in expository writing. Loving to write and having been told I showed "potential," I looked forward to the course. Our first paper was supposed to be written over a semester break and sent in before our return. As I sealed the envelope, I was half convinced it would come back with rave reviews and red-pencil notes indicating that it should immediately be sent to *The New Yorker* or *Harper's* for publication. But even if it wasn't published, it just had to be an A.

Well, I got a C. And to my chagrin, somebody else's paper was read in class instead of mine. Assigned to write a paper a week, each demonstrating a different mode of rhetoric, I quickly determined that my next paper would be the best in the class no matter what. All week long I pored over a first, second, third, and final draft to remove any potential flaws.

That paper too returned with a depressing C. So did the next. For each of ten agonizing weeks I received a C. The frustrating part of it was that I couldn't figure out why all my classmates were doing so well. Their papers seemed lucid but not particularly profound. My massive paragraphs and perfectly sculptured sentences were overlooked despite all the work. I knew the others couldn't be putting in all the time I did, and yet hard work brought no results. It was a great deal like my diabetes. I had plenty of intensity there too, but kept ending up with problems.

Toward the end of the term we were assigned to write a comparison/contrast. I decide to compare and contrast Hemingway and Fitzgerald. After killing myself on the serious paper, I decided, as a lark, to figure out the percentages of adverbs, adjectives, nouns, and pronouns each had used in the opening paragraphs of his novels. Then I decided to include a graph on the final page of my paper that connected percentage points with colorful lines, like a corporate sales report. Finally, figuring I had nothing to lose, I wrote the following sentence beneath the graph: "The above chart reveals parts of speech percentages used by Mr. Hemingway and Mr. Fitzgerald. So far as I can tell, it means absolutely nothing at all."

I was so angry about my string of C's that if the paper had come back saying my cynicism was entirely out of line, I don't think I would have cared. An F would be better than a nondescript C. When I walked into class the following Monday, there was my paper. All eight pages, including the graph with its glib slur, had been reproduced. We spent almost twenty minutes looking over the solid, well-constructed, and boring paragraphs. Then Dr. Ray asked everyone to turn to the last page.

"Read that final sentence," he said with a half-smile. My heart sank. I was convinced everyone would laugh, and so they did.

"That, Mr. Pray,", said Dr. Ray, "is one of the very few sentences you've actually written this entire term. And that is a fine sentence."

I walked out of the class pleased with my B, but curious. All those sentences I'd so carefully tried to fix were so studied they didn't have much life. In an offhand moment, I'd written a sarcastic sentence because there was something I wanted to say. Dr. Ray was a fine teacher. He didn't cater. He knew I had to work less on writing and more on simply being myself. One would lead to the other, but it wouldn't always work the other way around.

So it was with my diabetes. So much time had been spent trying to cut the deck that I wasn't getting to the game. I couldn't believe I had gained all that weight, that my exercise was twice as intense but not part of any routine. It was a though the three horses of diabetes were running every which way without a sense of direction. And hard as it was to believe, I had actually tried to clobber another person because he reminded me of myself.

What Dr. Ray had told me about my writing could have been said about my life. What was true for my life was true for my diabetes. Those are the lessons I could have learned if I'd had ears to hear and eyes to see. But I didn't. To me, life and disease couldn't possibly be one and the same.

25 ✦ BUCKHORN

It was August again. The confusing summer term was finished, and it was time to head off for a job. Beloit had a plan that let students practice what they'd learned, and when I asked what jobs might be available, I was told about the Buckhorn Children's Center in the mountains of eastern Kentucky.

Buckhorn was a town of fewer than a hundred people in the middle of coal country. From what the placement office said, the stories about blinking and maybe missing it were true. The Center was run by the Presbyterian Church, and boarded a variety of kids. Some were troubled, some were orphans, some couldn't stay with their families. Thoughts of Appalachia ran through my imagination like black-and-white movies of the Depression, and the more I heard the more I wanted to go.

I was excited about the chance to become a teacher. Teaching implied a personal responsibility to others that reinforced my determination to keep diabetes from posing any problems. Letting myself down was one thing, but letting others down would be a major reverse. Diabetes had never been a problem, and now it couldn't be.

In an odd way, working at Buckhorn helped me get Vietnam out of my system. As a diabetic, I was ineligible for the draft everyone else was trying to avoid. As Vietnam grew into a nightmare no matter whose side you were on, being labeled 4-F from the beginning was a mixed blessing. It provided a troubling sanctuary from the concerns and personal decisions that touched my generation, and left a desire to build the new era in my own way.

Getting to Buckhorn challenged my pledges to keep diabetes in the background. I loved to travel, but my system didn't. Traveling meant trusting somebody else's schedule. If the plane was late, if by accident the lunch served was inadequate, or if an economy flight skipped lunch entirely and only handed out peanut packets, I'd be in a mess. The thought of applying in advance for the special diabetic meals would have been like allowing someone else to clip my nails. It was a nice service, but not for me.

I caught a plane in Chicago bound for Lexington. On board there were about sixty empty seats and two chatting stewardesses. I chose a seat, sat down, and waited for some more passengers. Two eventually showed up and we taxied out for the takeoff. During the flight, one of the stewardesses offered me drinks in the same tone she would have used if there had been sixty passengers on the plane. Thank you, I said, going along with the game. You're welcome, she said ever so politely with a slight Southern accent. I should have remembered how sensations of irony can forewarn of a reaction, because fifteen minutes later, in the clear skies over Indiana, I began to slip. The stewardesses had an ample supply of Cokes and nothing to do, but I didn't want to disturb them. That was the second warning: I didn't feel I could or should ask for help.

By the time the plane landed, my vision was beginning to blur. I walked straight to the lunch counter in the small Lexington airport and ordered a large Coke and a cheeseburger platter. Trying not to slur my words, I asked the waitress to kindly bring the Coke first. In the South, I'd heard, everything happened at its own leisurely pace. She more than lived up to the tradition as she moved ever so slowly down the counter line, chatting with customers, picking up checks, counting tips, and taking her time.

I glanced over to the candy bars at the cash register, trying to determine if I had the strength to make it over there and buy one. I finally decided it was safer to just save whatever energy I had by hanging on at my seat until she brought the Coke. Eventually she did, and I downed it in about two seconds flat. Then came the cheeseburger. I devoured it, and the fries, and the pickle, the chips, and all the cole slaw that came with the platter.

It is very difficult in the midst of a reaction to avoid eating too much. After all, food ensures a return to safety, so it is natural to just keep eating until the food takes effect. By the time it does, however, there is frequently a bounce-back that shoots blood sugar levels far higher than they should be.

During a reaction, the body searches for its hidden stores of sugar. Eventually, unless there are convulsions that lead to choking or a diabetic has intentionally taken a suicidal amount of insulin, enough sugar is released to end a reaction. The problem is that the body then keeps on releasing sugars for some time. This process, known as the Somogyi effect, means that there are really two rescue missions at work. Food does its job and the body does its own internal work for up to ten hours. The onslaught of sugar produces a sudden and sickening change in direction that can throw control off kilter for several days. The lack of control can then set the stage for another reaction, as had happened to me in France.

It is essential, therefore, not to eat too much food when on the brink of or in the midst of a reaction. One glass of orange juice is usually plenty. The difficulty is that it takes a few minutes for the emergency glass of juice to take effect. During those minutes, the desire to keep eating and drinking is as strong as the desire for survival. The Greeks said moderation is a virtue. But the Greeks never sit in the Lexington airport with trembling hands waiting for a Coke and greasy cheeseburger to take effect.

After a restless night in a cheap hotel, I had a strange breakfast of biscuits and gravy before boarding the bus for Hazard. We quickly crossed the rolling Kentucky plains and, moving from a highway to a small road, entered the soft green Appalachians. They weren't like the dramatic hard-rock mountains I'd known out West. These hills were covered with deciduous trees, and in the valleys were creeks and small towns. Beside the road were houses, each with a porch that seemed filled with people. Kudzu vines cascaded down the sides of hills and moved up the telephone poles and street signs. For the first time I saw coal in thin seams along the road cuts. It was an altogether new world, and I couldn't have been happier.

The Center's director met me and a co-worker at the Hazard bus depot about five thirty. He had read on my application that I was diabetic, but didn't ask a thing about it. I asked him how long a drive it would be to the Center, trying to figure out when we would eat. He must have picked up the hint, because we soon pulled into a gas station/café for dinner. Still trying to steady myself from the Lexington reaction, I ate mostly meat and salad, thinking carbohydrates would worsen an already high blood sugar.

Although I'd had a good many jobs before, this was the first that couldn't be considered an "odd job." My specific mission was to teach ten or so kids everything I could about science and math. When I mentioned that I wasn't much at math, the director smiled and told me the first thing to do was to meet the kids and get a feeling for the Center.

The next morning I was sitting in his office talking about the kids, the rules, and the nature of my job when I simply up and keeled over. It was the only day reaction I've ever had that I couldn't feel coming on. There were no signs, no warnings, and it let me understand the terror many diabetics have when they've lost their ability to foretell a reaction. Why it happened to me that morning I don't know. It was probably a mixture of the traveling, the Somogyi rebound, the string of small reactions I'd been having that August, and the emotion of the moment. When I fell, I gashed my forehead at the hairline.

The director and an aide lifted me into the car and asked the nurse to drive me to the hospital in Hazard. Halfway there, I woke up wondering what had happened. I didn't need to spend a day in the hospital, but that is where she put me despite my protests. A doctor and I adjusted my insulin dose, and the next day I went back to the job I really hadn't even started. The kids all knew something had happened because they could see the gash and stitches.

"What happened, Mr. Larry?" they asked. I briefly told them about diabetes and then tried to change the subject as fast as possible. Little did I realize that good teaching is anything but a one-way street, and that the way we all shared our strengths and handled our weaknesses brought us together. Like me, the kids were just different enough to feel very different. Just the way Appalachia was supposed to "fit in" with the rest of society, these kids were supposed to eventually "fit in" with the public-school kids across the street. Although we couldn't help feeling we were the ones out of step, we developed a pride as we shared our lives.

Some of the kids were retarded, some disturbed; others had no place to go and no one to take them. One was convinced that almost any visitor to the Center might adopt him and take him home. One could write his name but couldn't write anything else. He could take apart any engine in the state of Kentucky, but he couldn't write. Another wouldn't talk. When we rehearsed our Christmas play he never said a word. But on that final night, silent Dan spoke with a loud and clear voice that surprised and moved everyone, including himself. One was so tough he had to learn to laugh. One so wild he had to slow down; one so in love with any young man she had to learn to care for herself. These kids forged my foundation as a teacher.

We plunged into science and math head first and developed the Buckhorn Zoo. It included two goldfish, one parakeet, a toad, a spare white rat from the University of Kentucky (we said that we needed one for research), and last but not least, a possum. The kids told me that the best way to catch a possum was to find one at the dump some night and give it a big kick. Once scared, the possum would play possum and could be picked up without any difficulty.

We built a complicated cardboard maze for our rat and watched it figure out every obstacle we could put in its way. We made sure the bird didn't fly away, and after a week of watching the possum refuse to eat we tried to get him (or her) to leave. He (or she) wouldn't. Finally we put the cage outside and left the door wide open all night. By morning, our possum had vanished.

I disliked leaving the kids before Christmas. We came from different starting points, but we all had our problems. Education meant growing up with them instead of against them. In a way, my three stitches and bobtail-like wisp of hair that grew out all fall long was a reminder of the diabetes that had landed me in the hospital and deepened my bond with the kids. Since then, there have been plenty of other reminders of the unforgettable Appalachian fall, because it was through Buckhorn that I met my wife.

26 • LOVE STORY

It is with trepidation that I write the love story of a diabetic. It seems farfetched even to think that diabetes has anything to do with love stories, and to assume that there might be some kind of pattern to the love lives of diabetics seems fanciful and bizarre, to say the least.

So, to the Don Juans of diabetes, to those who somewhere along the line have fallen in love with a diabetic, to the shy and the bold, to the young diabetics who may swear on a stack of Bibles they'll never get married or fall in love no matter what, I apologize. I can only say that contrary to my expectations, I found that love stories and diabetes do in fact go hand in hand. More than I thought possible, each directly influenced the future of the other. Falling in love was an interlude of lasting implications. In the short run, it evened out my control. In the long run, the relationship with another person helped guide and push me toward acceptance.

That there would ever be a love story to write about required an about-face. I believed as a young teen-ager that any notion even approaching the idea of marriage would be out of the question. My decision had nothing to do with not caring for girls, because that wasn't the case at all. The problem was a matter of cold-blooded logic. Love implied marriage, marriage implied children, and diabetes was an inherited disease. That meant our children might one day be diabetic. The thought of passing on my disease wasn't appealing, to say the least. And there was a more ominous reason that gnawed at my social confidence. If it weren't for insulin, I wouldn't even be alive. So what right did I have to pass on diabetes when Mother Nature wouldn't have had me around in the first place?

It was the kind of logic that was so right it just had to be wrong. But it seemed unassailable, and those thoughts carried the day for a good many years. I loved life as much then as I do now, and while sometimes lonely, I didn't consider myself a brooding or depressed person in the least. There were plenty of people who made contributions without getting married and having kids, I said to myself, and that was the way I determined with adolescent conviction I'd some- day be.

It is amazing how easily adults forget those kinds of feelings. After I'd been married ten years and we had three of our four kids, I spoke with a diabetic girl who was having great difficulty accepting her dia- betes. She had many talents and the support of her family, but her life seemed like a series of new starts. Each showed potential, but none pointed in a firm direction. At age seventeen, she had one overriding purpose: not to be diabetic. To prove the point, she had simply stopped taking her shots.

"Think about your future," I said as the extent of her denial and magical thinking finally hit home. "Someday you'll be married and have a family and a career of your own. Don't do yourself in when someday people will depend on you." Her eyes began to tear up, but her expression hardened.

"Do you see yourself getting married someday?" I asked, thinking for some reason her answer would be yes.

"No," she said in broken anger with the tears now streaming. My first reaction was disbelief. Then it hit me. When I too was seventeen, eighteen, nineteen, and even twenty, I had seen myself much the same way. How can you pass on or share something you want to deny? How can you expect others to love you when you're trying to reject yourself? Since diabetes had no cure, and since acceptance seemed an almost ludicrous thought, she had taken herself out of the running.

"Stay with it," I said, not knowing quite what else to say. "I felt the same way when I was seventeen. Believe it or not, you'll get past these barriers if you'll give yourself a chance. Take it one day at a time, and don't forget that you never know what may happen."

For me, the first break in my watertight denial came when I met the girl who took my place at Buckhorn. I'd been back at Beloit for a few weeks when some friends I'd met at Buckhorn came for a visit. They'd asked if they couldn't bring her along. I told them that it would be all right with me if they really needed the company on their long drive. I didn't know they'd told her about the Buckhorn Zoo and our play and had shown her some poems I'd written on lonely Kentucky nights.

They arrived about seven and parked their car on the street alongside my window. I looked out, saw them wave, and grabbed a sweater. Halfway out the door I was still trying to get the sweater on and had the arms all confused with the neck.

"Hello," they said with a laugh as they watched me try to arrange myself into some semblance of order.

"Hello yourself," I said.

"This is Connie."

"Hi," I said, scarcely giving her the time of day. They unpacked the car and came into my tiny room. We spent much of the night talking about the Center and its kids, trying to reconcile the vast difference between college academics and people's real lives. Throughout the talk I kept glancing at Connie. She hadn't been at Buckhorn long, but she too had fallen in love with the kids and the sure rhythms of Appalachia. It turned out her family came from there, that she was part Cherokee, that the mountains I'd known in the fall would be still more beautiful in the spring. She had dark hair and hazel eyes. Hazel is one of those colors that one never quite finds on charts, but once seen it stays with you. So it was with her.

My friends had told her I was diabetic before we met. Realizing how important meals were, we all met for a solid breakfast the next morning. I found myself interested in Buckhorn and curiously enraptured with Connie. We lingered over several last cups of coffee in a greasy-spoon café, and hated to see the brief visit come to an end. The matchmakers must have been pleased.

Three weeks later I found it made a lot of sense to take a weekend break from the rigors of academic life and pay a visit to eastern Kentucky. We took a good many walks up the hollows, stole a good many kisses, and to my surprise and delight knew we were falling in love.

Diabetes' first intrusion came by accident. We were at our friends' cottage. It was about nine o'clock, and I had just left the group to take my shot in the back room. I didn't tell anybody where I was going, as good manners and common sense had always made taking a shot a private affair. I then heard a knock at the front door and a girl's voice. For some reason, Connie did not want this girl to know she was there. To avoid her, she suddenly came into the back room just as I was in the middle of drawing my insulin. She watched me as I finished, and then, figuring the cat was out of the bag, I went ahead and gave myself a quick jab into my arm. To my surprise, it wasn't embarrassing. She hadn't recoiled as I thought she might. I wondered for just a second if she thought I was brave, and then realized what a juvenile thought that was. We waited for the other girl to leave, and then returned to the front room.

With other girlfriends, both potential and real, I had kept diabetes a secret. One relationship had more or less ended when I mentioned my diabetes after our first few encounters. I thought the girl might be interested in knowing about it, but quite the opposite was true. Connie's stability in knowing I was diabetic was as reassuring as her presence was pleasing. I never realized until a good deal later that she had to disregard some frightening advice and hang on to her instincts.

"After I first met you," she said as we talked about our romance, "I was with Maggie Wilder, the Center's nurse. She was an old nurse who had worked way back in the hills for years and years. I was really smitten and was sure you were the one I was going to end up with.

"I was talking with her about that when all of a sudden she sat me down and gave me this long lecture about her husband. It turned out he had been diabetic for years, and ended up dying young and leaving her a widow. She still hadn't quite gotten over it.

"She asked if I was prepared for that and for all the complications. She went into this long, gory sermon about all the awful things that could happen to a diabetic. I was just crushed. I hadn't even thought about those things. But that's the kind of sermon I got from several people. They weren't saying to steer clear, but there was a doomsday feeling to it."

"Well," I said, "I didn't exactly help things when I conked out that

143

day. Maggie was the nurse who took me to the hospital. That trip must have brought back all kinds of memories for her."

It's ironic that Maggie knew more about the complications of diabetes than I did at that stage of the game. I didn't know she'd had a diabetic husband. Perhaps she assumed I knew about all the problems. Or maybe she didn't want to be the bearer of bad news. In any case, thank heaven Connie put her fears to the side.

"From the beginning," she said, "your diabetes was more or less out in the open. In fact, I was surprised because your friends had said something about your being secretive about it. You didn't talk about how you felt as a diabetic, but neither did you hide your shot."

The truth was, I didn't hide it from her. And just as she figured she'd end up with me, I figured I'd end up with her. Entertaining that thought brought a mixture of amazement, joy, and more than a touch of disbelief. It took us more than a year of ups and downs to test it all out. It was, to say it simply, a love story.

27 ✦ *TRANSITIONS*

On my way to Maine for a summer job a year and a half later, I stopped off in Michigan to see Connie. I'd been a newspaper reporter in Montana and a graduate student in Iowa during our year-long estrangement. We had only one day to mend fences, but that was all we needed. When she came to visit me at the end of the summer, I romantically planned that we'd climb a mountain together and then I'd ask her to marry me at the top.

"Larry," she said as we sat in a meadow overlooking the mountain the day before the climb, "do you think we should get married?"

"Yes," I said, irked that she had stolen my thunder.

"Good," she said, and that was the end of that. The day after Christmas we were married at my parents' home in Wisconsin. Like most marriages, it was filled with the vows and hopes of a new beginning. For my parents, it marked letting go of both a son and the emotional guardianship of his disease.

It may seem strange that that hadn't already happened. After all, I'd been out on my own for six years. But more than any of us realized, diabetes had a hold on our relationship. Like all families, we had a mental picture of the kind of family and people we wanted to be. Diabetes was a hitch in the scheme of things that jarred our ideals and wouldn't go away.

"Our relationship," said my mother as we talked about it with the clarity of hindsight, "had a burden on it that wouldn't have been there if you hadn't been diabetic. The very nature of diabetes, with its constant vigilance, doesn't make it something you can forget at any moment. Night, morning, and noon it's always present. It wasn't until you got married that I could begin to put it all behind me. It wasn't until then that I knew my job was done."

There was a second side to my mother's letting go. Just as diabetes once made me doubt the kind of son I had been, it made her doubt the kind of mother she had been. She wanted me relieved of the hovering mother she considered herself to be. I had never seen her that way, but my perceptions weren't important; those were her feelings. While there was support and love, it was as though we needed the distance marriage could give to see things clearly. Her letting go gave Connie the first inkling of what diabetes' impact on our family life had really been.

"On the day of our wedding," she said, "your mother and I were cooking together. In the midst of a chat she said something like 'Well, now he's yours.' It struck me that she was talking about your diabetes as much or more than you as a person. I could feel her turning over a lot of her pressure and worry. It felt as though she'd been a servant to the diabetes for so long. But I knew in the same instant that I wouldn't be like your mother, and that I shouldn't carry it the way she had."

Exactly what her approach should be was something neither of us worried about much. We both simply assumed everything would work out. With the pride of a new husband I was confident she'd never have to worry about me. We worked out our wedding ceremony to include Kahlil Gibran's poem on marriage. Share your lives, he admonished, but be careful to leave distances between you. What those distances needed to be took us both some time to discover. And frankly, distance was the furthest thing from our minds as we finished our wedding dinner, climbed into a used VW, and headed off into the night in the midst of a December blizzard.

Our plan was to travel across Canada and down through New England interviewing at schools for a teaching position on our way to Baltimore, where I was a graduate student at Johns Hopkins. Once we arrived, we settled into a small row house. It wasn't much, but then it didn't need to be. There was no room for an office, so I set one up in the large bathroom and used the tub as a wastepaper basket. Our kitchen was so small we couldn't even open the oven door, and the proverbial orange crates did indeed make fine shelves.

One night as we did our homework for this book, Dick Evans came over for dinner and we explored marriage and diabetes.

"When we first got married," said Connie, thinking back on our early days together, "I remember making three fine meals a day, shopping for wholesome vegetables in Baltimore's Lexington Market, and making sure everything was right. It was a very romantic period, but it also had a gamelike quality to it. We kept your diabetes mostly private. I had to learn what you already knew, and remember your taking time to teach me about food and exercise. I knew the danger signs of reactions, but your teaching gave me an understanding about what went into diabetes as a whole."

"It surprised me," I said, "how much our marriage evened out my control. I still had some close calls, but that's just part of being diabetic. Even after eleven years, you've never seen me pass out from a reaction. I think that's the result of our marriage."

"It doesn't surprise me that your violent reactions stopped once you got married," said Dick. "Marriage can be a stabilizing influence. Statistics indicate that people have fewer accidents and get less sick when they are married. They're less depressed, too.

"Marriage is an escape from the authority of your parents, even if you haven't been living with them. Now you are on your own. Now you're a parent, or a potential parent, yourself. As long as you aren't overly dependent on each other as a couple, it can provide a stable base."

"It gave me a sense of belonging," I said. "That is a very important feeling."

"Belonging, without being overdominated, is a tricky but crucial factor in marriage. And the importance is magnified for a diabetic," said Dick. "It sounds to me as though you both stumbled and worked your way through to that kind of relationship."

"It wasn't simple," said Connie to me. "I was more aware of your diabetes than you probably realized. The one time I got scared was on a day we were taking a walk through Baltimore and as usual, we didn't have any money. You went into a reaction and I ran into this

147

little dive to ask for a glass of juice. I couldn't even pay for it, so I just demanded it. You recovered, but I remember the terror of watching you slip, knowing that we had no money and wondering what I was going to do. That incident has always stayed with me, and set the tone for a while."

"I'd forgotten all about that," I said.

"Well, I didn't want to embarrass you. I'd make sure you were okay at the vulnerable times and tried to anticipate what you'd need. To you it probably seemed as if an orange just suddenly appeared when you needed a snack. It really got tough once you started teaching and classes ran late, or meetings ran longer than planned. You were probably in control of the situation, but I'd worry anyway and would try to figure out how to get that orange to you without your being embarrassed and without my feeling like your maid."

As she spoke I remembered the neatly folded notes I'd sometimes get at noon saying a snack was available if needed. Ninety-nine percent of the time I didn't need the orange, but not wanting to embarrass Connie, I didn't have the heart to tell her.

"If you had worried openly about Larry's diabetes every minute," Dick said to Connie, "it could have become a kind of scapegoat in your marriage. You might have become a martyr, and that wouldn't have been good for either one of you."

"The one thing I never did say," said Connie, "or even felt much, was 'If only you knew what I went through getting that orange to appear at the right time!' I'd seen some families where that had happened, and I didn't want to be like them."

"It was a good thing you weren't," said Dick. "Because if you were, you would have become more mother and less wife to Larry."

"But I still had to wean myself away from his diabetes," Connie replied. "There came a certain point when I realized I couldn't always be there. And I saw how easy it would be for me to build myself into a kind of protector-provider. I knew if I let that escalate too much, it would get out of control for both of us. I saw that that wouldn't help him at all. When I was trying to anticipate everything in advance, that really took its toll."

"Well," said Dick, "marriage should provide someone who knows you as a peer rather than as a parent. That is why it was so important for you to see that diabetes was Larry's challenge and not yours. If you hadn't done that, you would have really interfered with the acceptance process. The same is true for parents of juvenile diabetics. If the parents take on too much, they'll get in the way. That is not to say that a parent isn't going to develop and keep a special kind of vigilance, much as Larry's mother did. But too much of anything is a bad thing, especially when it prevents someone from taking care of himself."

Determining the lines of responsibility is a challenge every family touched by diabetes must face. Each family must set its own timetable for letting go, and while there isn't a "right" way to do it, the consequences of not letting go can be serious. Families in which the parents carry the burden of diabetes more than their child wind up with serious problems. It would have been so easy for my parents to step in and bail me out when I labored over my slow shots way back in the third grade. Their coming to my rescue might have given them the reassuring feeling of being helpers, but it would have been the wrong thing to do.

"During that first year of our marriage," said Connie after we'd cleared away the dishes and sat down for some coffee with Dick, "I got a real feel for the two sides of your diabetes. It was almost as though diabetes was a silent opponent in a boxing ring, and you were fighting with it all the time. That fight kept going and going just beneath the surface until you finally came to terms with diabetes in your life. It was as though you were angry, and kept trying to push it all down."

"I didn't want diabetes to interfere with the family," I said. "I was working as best I could to keep things under control."

"That's the whole willpower phase," said Dick. "You had to learn that conquering something and accepting it are two different things."

"I felt you were in a race with yourself," said Connie. "And I knew there was a fear. It was almost as if you were saying, 'I don't have long' without your really saying it. I think that is where a lot of your intensity came from."

"That sense of urgency has some pluses with it," said Dick. "You know, F.D.R. was kind of a goof-off before he had polio. Then he realized what life was really about and he grew up in a hurry. It changed him. You strike me as the kind of person who wants to do something you really believe in. I wonder how much that is a result of your diabetes."

"Maybe that is a trait of the sixties generation," I said.

"Maybe it is. But your diabetes may have helped you reckon at an earlier age with what you wanted to do. Everybody, even the most 'successful' people, eventually should come to terms with what they want to leave behind them. Most of us do it as we get older. Look at the number of people who want to get out of the so-called rat race. They go from high-paying jobs in New York City to buying a mom-and-pop grocery store in Vermont, or something like that.

"I'm not trying to say there aren't many ways to define meaning in life. Making a lot of money, helping society, trying to leave something behind all may or may not be fulfilling. But eventually success has to be measured from within, and that realization is avoided until later in life by many people.

"I suspect there was a greater urgency on your part, because you had to come to terms with your mortality quicker than most because of your diabetes. I think that's what Connie sensed when you first got married."

"I suppose that's true," I said. "I haven't really banked on seeing much old age. I haven't had any complications after these twenty-seven years, but that's no guarantee something won't happen. If anything, that sense of urgency has inspired me."

The first year of our marriage was a curious year. For both Connie and me, it was a time of learning how to share our lives. As we better realized what we could and could not do, we began to grow up, and just as it should have, the honeymoon came to an end.

28 ⬧ TEACHING

Looking for a job in the spring of 1971 reminded me that there were, of course, some jobs a diabetic simply couldn't have. We couldn't, for example, be airline pilots, astronauts, candy tasters, or hold down jobs with constantly changing schedules. Unfortunately, for some diabetics, the limitations went still further. My father had once said that two problems that came with diabetes were job discrimination and expensive life insurance. You may have to be careful, he told me, because some employers think diabetes is really a lot worse than it is.

But the sword could cut the other way as well. Not only might organizations discriminate against diabetics: diabetics might discriminate against themselves as well. The worse their acceptance, the more impossible a job they'd choose, and a checkmate would naturally ensue.

One teen-ager who wouldn't take his shots and had several times come dangerously close to not making it told me one evening he wanted to be an airline pilot.

"You realize," I said, "you have chosen the one sure job you absolutely cannot have. Even if you were the best diabetic in the world and had all the nerves of an ace pilot, you still couldn't have that job."

He shrugged his shoulders as if to say he knew but still wanted to be a pilot. His denial of diabetes had crossed over into a denial of his future. His parents looked on, naturally scared to death and not knowing what to do. They had ended up with most of his responsibility. The more they tried to get him to take care of himself, the more he rebelled. When they turned the other way, he wouldn't take his shots. And so it went.

Another diabetic kept waiting and waiting for the day his diabetes would get under control, and *then* he would be able to launch a career in earnest. The day was always in the future. For him the idea of professional responsibility required a kind of perfection, and not being perfect gave him a curious kind of escape.

In my case, I wanted to teach and, just as I had at Buckhorn, figured diabetes could be kept separate from my profession. Our honeymoon interviews hadn't panned out, so I wrote a second batch of letters to schools. Finally, a letter from Maine came, asking me to come up for an interview at the Hyde School in Bath. Within several days we were in the car and heading for the State of Maine.

I will never forget the sincerity of the kids we met that March day. In the gracious mansion of a former shipbuilder were a hundred and ten kids excited as they could be about their education. This is our school, they seemed to say. It may or may not be the greatest school in the world, but it's unique, has a vision of what education should be, and it is our school. The kids told me Hyde stressed attitudes as well as achievements, and that everyone had an oar to pull. It wasn't a free school; it wasn't a military school. It simply challenged everyone to grow, and had been accredited for the teaching of character. From the looks on their faces and the way they all talked about a new philosophy of education, I believed them.

Diabetes didn't surface in the interview, but I wouldn't have felt right not bringing it up with the Headmaster, Joe Gauld.

"Listen," I said as we finished up, "there is one thing I haven't mentioned. I am a diabetic. I haven't had any problems with it, I am in good control of myself, and it has been several years since I've had a serious reaction. But I did think you should know."

"No problem," he said with a big smile. "I appreciate your bringing it up. We have another teacher here who is diabetic. He is six feet four and it hasn't been a problem for him."

"Thanks," I said, wondering why he thought size had anything to do with diabetes. When he offered me the job that afternoon, I told him I'd like to think it over. Half an hour later I found him at the tennis court and told him I wanted to come aboard starting in the fall.

In Baltimore, our bathtub had been my wastepaper basket. In Bath, our tub became our kitchen sink in a tiny apartment. But teaching was just as challenging and exciting as I had known it would be. Teaching "growth" and character development as well as academic competence put education in a whole new light. Just as the kids were expected to challenge their courage, curiosity, and leadership, so were the faculty supposed to challenge theirs. Telling a young person to grow up is easy. Having such a statement take root in a young person's imagination is quite another thing. Wisdom and advice must be transmitted in a way that inspires each individual. A kid may know his fears and talk around them, but may need a wrestling mat to find his courage. A teacher can preach honesty, but must then search his own integrity. Although these searches are precisely what one needs, they also reach deeper than one sometimes wants to go. In my case, trying to teach character brought my rejection of diabetes sharply into focus.

Just before Thanksgiving vacation, we were having a school meeting. At the Hyde School there was a double stairway in the central hallway with Greek columns on both sides. An elegant place, it was the spiritual heart of our school. Whenever there were problems, evaluations, spontaneous concerns, or tedious talks about character education, we met there on the steps. The problem this time was standards. No smoking or drugs were allowed at the school, and the ethic behind the standards was very real. If someone was caught or turned himself in, it became a matter of conscience and trust. But vacations were quite another matter.

"I don't see," said one kid, "why we can't have a little freedom over the vacations. School rules shouldn't follow us all the time!"

"So," said a faculty member. "So that's all this place means to you. Character is something you can turn on and off whenever you want to, is that it?"

The argument got hot and heavy. It was the same kind of argument I'd heard running through my own mind for many years. The thought of being a picture-perfect diabetic who followed all the rules was hardly inspiring. But that didn't mean I should go off the deep end. Unable to live with either approach all the time, I kept switching. For both me and the school there was a paradox in there some-where that was hard to resolve. At one point in the argument, all six feet four inches of the other diabetic faculty member stood up to speak.

"Listen," he said with a good deal of emotion in his voice. "Some of you ought to find out what standards are all about! Look at Mr. Pray, for example. He's got to run, take two shots every day, and watch his diet exactly because he's diabetic. If he stops doing any one of those those things he'll die! So grow up, will you!"

The whole school quieted down in an instant, and I felt all the eyes turn toward me as the blood ran to my face. There have been few times in my life I felt as angry as I did that morning eleven years ago. If I'd been standing near him I would have come close to taking a wild swing and decking him as best I could. As it was, I glared across the foyer and tried to let him know he had done something terrible. Never before had my diabetes been an open book for public record. The personal and professional lines that shouldn't have been crossed had not only been crossed, they had been ignored and erased. It was a shattering experience.

As soon as the school meeting broke up, I went straight over to Jeff and told him he had had no right to say what he did. He apologized, surprised that he had revealed a secret. To Jeff, diabetes was an open subject. He and I went running every morning at six through the streets of Bath. When desserts were served at the school, our waiter always brought us each an apple and a slice of cheese. On those mornings we had French toast, the chef prepared us each a slice of meat. As far as everyone could see, my condition was nothing partic-ularly unusual. In an ironic way, what I was afraid of their knowing was really something I was afraid of admitting to myself. To the kids, diabetes was nothing to be ashamed of. But to me, it was unaccept-able. After the incident with Jeff, Connie saw the conflict better than anyone else.

"That was the first time I knew diabetes was bigger than you or me. I knew after that I had to back out entirely. Your anger was far bigger than the incident. In a way, it was the first time I saw the full extent of your anger as a diabetic. You were furious to see your dia-betes revealed and to have it tied to your growth. Part of what made you mad was that you realized you couldn't divide your personal and professional lives. You had to merge them or go backwards, and it really made you mad.

"The odd thing was, your diabetes looked great to a lot of people. But to me, and to you after that incident, it was almost a life force you were fighting. It really weighed you down back then. And the more it weighed you down, the more you tried to conquer it. It was as though you were trying to prove yourself.

"I was so embarrassed for you at that meeting, but in another way I was relieved."

It is hard to believe, but throughout practically all my years before acceptance, if someone had asked me if I was angry about diabetes, I would have answered no. It would have been an honest answer. The idea of getting angry at a disease had always seemed selfish. The adage about the man who felt sorry for himself because he had no shoes and then met a man who had no feet had always carried a lot of weight. After Jeff's revelation, I came face to face with the anger I'd so long denied.

To make matters worse, not only had he revealed my diabetes, he had told the school what an exemplary diabetic I was, when I knew that wasn't anywhere near the truth. I didn't count calories, played catch-up ball much of the time, and was reluctant to give in to the meticulous care I knew so well how to do. It didn't matter that compared with others I was in fine shape, and that "the rest of my life" was moving right along. Now that he had spoken, I had to both clean up my act and admit to being diabetic.

Then the full implications hit me. I was a professional in a school that asked for openness and yet the truth made me seethe. Why was I so angry? All Jeff had done was let an obvious cat out of the bag. We were, after all, trying to teach kids that the truth should inform their lives. Could I then continue to deny the truth about myself? And if my diabetes wasn't all that exemplary, shouldn't I simply redouble my efforts to do something about it? The more I thought about it, the more I knew my anger was misplaced. I would eventually have to come to terms with the truth. My safe and private boundaries would never lead to acceptance, and could no longer contain my disease.

29 • COMPLICATIONS

Now that my diabetes was a public instead of a private disease, I wanted to become the best diabetic and the best teacher I could possibly be. Both were tall orders. Work in a boarding school can be a very intense experience, because the teaching never really ends. Morning, noon, and night the kids' lives became our lives. There was always another student to see, another paper to grade, the next track meet to prepare for, the next unexpected personal challenge in the life of a youngster. It seemed as though everybody did everything and it all happened at once. Connie and I both thrived on the intensity and wondered how on earth we'd ever keep up.

During my first evaluation by the kids, I could scarcely believe it when they said they admired and respected my teaching. I was so convinced they were going to nail me for my shortcomings that their praise left me tearfully overwhelmed. After the evaluation, the faculty congratulated me profusely. When we met as a faculty, however, the Headmaster saw it differently.

"Don't let that happen again," he said. "You can't afford such a difference between your expectations and the kids' evaluations. You need to take more confidence in what you do."

I wasn't sure just what he meant, but as I look back on it now I can see that my uncertainties about diabetes had crossed over into my professional life. It's not that I thought about diabetes each and every moment, because I didn't. But whenever I was caught off guard with too low or too high a blood sugar, or whenever I felt like breaking the rules in spite of myself, it reared its head as an unwelcome but persistent reminder of my Achilles' heel. In my mind, I would always be on the short end of the stick until I found the willpower to conquer and master my diabetes.

After several years, however, I felt myself beginning to wear out. Some of it was the pace of things. Between coaching, teaching, trips on the ocean, and trying to hammer out a philosophy of education there wasn't much time (or so I said to myself) to manage diabetes. But even when things were calm, I didn't feel very well. I eventually went to the doctor in Bath, thinking that perhaps he could "do something." He thought insulin might be the culprit, so we changed to PZI. It did change things, but not for the better. It was almost as though the harder I tried the more problems I had. At that point, suspecting that something else was fundamentally wrong, I decided to enroll in Boston's famous Joslin Clinic. If there was anything wrong, I fully expected the Clinic could fix it and I'd emerge a new diabetic.

Despite my high hopes, walking into a hospital devoted to the care of diabetics spooked me at first. I remember heading across the lounge for the reception desk with a brisk and healthy stride that I hoped would disguise my diabetes, but the receptionist didn't seem to notice. In fact, my ego was thoroughly deflated when she methodically took my name and handed me a plastic container for a urine sample as though I were just like everyone else who came to the Clinic for an overhaul.

As I sat in the lounge waiting for things to be set up, I wondered who were the patients and who were simply visitors. Some of the cases were obvious. A young man in a wheelchair had evidently just had an amputation, and another had bandages over his eyes. It may have been my state of mind, but many people looked tired, as if diabetes had stolen their spirit. With the exception of the little kids who ran through the room, the atmosphere felt rather somber. For the first time, the potential complications of diabetes hit home.

I don't know why I had put off a serious investigation of the word "complications." My parents and doctors hadn't talked much about them, and perhaps it was just as well to keep fear at a distance. I had long known that the word "complications" meant more than it said.

But when I finally read in a pamphlet that half the juvenile diabetics die within twenty-five years of diagnosis, and that diabetes was listed by the American Diabetes Association as the third-leading cause of death in the United States, I wondered how I'd ever made it at all.

The flat-out statistics revealing the complications of diabetes are not difficult to find. Dick Evans showed me a chapter from the Scientific American book *Medicine* at one of our meetings. It described each problem I learned about at the Clinic with a lethal kind of certainty. "Atherosclerosis is the scourge of any diabetic," it reported. "It appears at an early age and becomes quite severe. Strokes are twice as frequent . . . and peripheral vascular problems are 50 to 100 times more frequent." In other words, diabetics have severe circulation problems. I'd known for many years that diabetics had heart problems, and used it as justification for my planned and erratic exercise.

"The diabetic is twenty-five times more prone to blindness and partial loss of vision than is the nondiabetic. The risk of developing cataracts is four to six times greater in the diabetic than in the nondiabetic, and the opacity develops at an earlier age. There is a two fold greater risk of glaucoma in diabetics. One in twenty of Insulin Dependent Diabetics becomes blind. About one in fifteen of Non Insulin Dependent Diabetics develops retinopathy, causing partial loss of sight, and one half of these become legally blind. Within three to five years after the onset of the disease, most diabetics develop vascular lesions, predominantly microaneurysms, and increased leakiness."

"Leaky" struck me as an amusing word for a not-so-amusing condition. When tiny veins in the eye break, the leaking blood can interrupt vision. That condition, called retinopathy, is a leading cause of blindness in the United States. Fortunately, this is one area where there is some hope. When it's found in time, doctors can zap the tiny veins with a laser beam to create a scar which more or less holds things together.

Kidney failure was still another problem. "Approximately one half of the Insulin Dependent Diabetics develop renal failure, usually after twenty to thirty years of the disease. Death results from myocardial infarction or congestive heart failure associated with uremia." Myocardial infarction, Dick told me, meant heart attack. Renal failure meant kidney failure, and that is why there was a dialysis unit at the Clinic.

Nerves came next. "Every diabetic has demonstrable neuropathic sequelae after several years of the disease. About one tenth develop significant symptoms, and one half of these have problems that are severe enough to be disabling." Neuropathic sequelae meant nerve damage. I'd always heard the bizarre story that diabetics might step on thumbtacks and not realize it until several days later when they accidentally discovered the tacks in their infected feet.

That sounded serious until I overheard four diabetic men talking one night about their problems with impotence. One was about to begin using a mechanical device, and while it was far better than nothing, I could feel the others wondering when and if they might have to come in for the same treatment. Diabetes, I had discovered, is also a "leading cause" of impotence. Because nerves don't regenerate, there was not much hope of finding a natural cure.

I have no idea what my reaction might be to losing my sight, or my limbs, or my capacity for sexual love. Speculation would probably be either overly heroic or maudlin. Those who face or have faced "complications" have emerged with their own stories of acceptance or denial. While I suspect the process isn't much different from coming to terms with diabetes in the first place, so far I haven't had to find out.

All of this made going to Joslin a little like making a pilgrimage to the headwaters of the Ganges or to Lourdes in hope of avoiding what the statistics said would happen. I should have remembered, but didn't, that the tough cases of complications were naturally at Joslin in increased numbers. I did keep telling myself that researchers were hard at work on finding a cure, and that there was no sense in brooding. The advice was sound, but not particularly comforting.

Because my bout with magical thinking had moved me away from assuming that thoughts could become things, I presumed my expectations wouldn't make too big a difference. The placebo effect that worked so well with some conditions wouldn't help much when it came to diabetes. After all, a diabetic injected with water instead of insulin would be in big trouble regardless of expectations.

One day, however, my sugar was far too high and I began to feel nauseated. I asked for and received a shot of quick-acting regular.

159

Within about five minutes I began to feel better. When I mentioned to the doctor that I could feel the sugar subsiding within me, he looked at me with a surprised expression.

"You know," he said, "there's no way the insulin could be working yet. It will take at least an hour or so before it makes much of a difference." I felt foolish, because as soon as he said it I knew he was right. And yet it really did feel as though my blood had begun to thin, so perhaps there was some truth in mind over matter after all.

"You know," said Dick as we talked about my first trip to Joslin, "I see two things in the way you reacted to being at Joslin. Your perception that some of the patients had more or less given up may have been fairly accurate. A good percentage of diabetics don't take care of themselves as far as exercise is concerned. Some tend to think of themselves as being less physically able, and then pamper themselves. The result is that they end up sedentary. They expect the worst to happen, and can sometimes fulfill their own expectations.

"The other thing is that being at Joslin interfered with your denial. Your going there was like an infantryman visiting a front-line hospital. He can say 'It ain't going to happen to me,' but when he sees other people it *has* happened to, it makes quite an impression."

"All of them said it wouldn't happen to them either," I added. "That's a good example of magical thinking, isn't it?"

"Right. Then he realizes he is just as vulnerable as they were."

"Going to Joslin was a real equalizer," I said. I had always wanted to be different from other diabetics. I wanted to be the first one to escape, the one who would never let it interfere, the one who would walk into Joslin and be mistaken for a nondiabetic. It was an uncomfortable but essential moment when I realized how much we were the same.

At the end of a class on the mechanics of diabetes, an older woman, rather hunched-over and wearing a drab gray overcoat despite the warmth of the room, approached the doctor.

"I know what you're saying," she said to him, "but my problem is that I can't get myself to do all these things. What should I do?"

"You just have to do it," he said in an annoyed voice as he packed his papers. How could he answer a nonspecific question?

"But," she pressed on.

160

"That's your problem," he said. I saw both the frustration of doctors whose patients don't follow the rules and the hurt on her face. He was correct that there was nothing he could give to help her accept her diabetes. And yet she had raised the kind of question that I am convinced lies, most rarely expressed, in most every diabetic's mind. Just asking it implies having the kind of problem diabetics aren't supposed to have. She wasn't the kind of person I wanted to identify with, but our search was undeniably the same.

When during my physical the doctor ran a dull blade across the bottom of my foot, I was so glad it tickled and felt cold that I could hardly stand it. Diabetics are probably the only people on earth who are actually pleased to feel the pain when they step on thumbtacks. When pictures were taken of my eyes, the examining doctor looked at me as though something were wrong.

"You have practically no traces of retinopathy," he said. "How did you do that?"

"I keep in shape," I said with a smug but delighted smile. In fact, keeping fit may or may not have had much to do with it. One of the kickers of complications is that while the statistics are accurate, who gets hit isn't entirely predictable. Although there is evidence that good control is the best line of defense, it can't guarantee a lack of complications. Some diabetics go for many years nearly unscathed, while others lose nerve function rather quickly.

During my stay the hospital staff watched my charts carefully, and devised a game plan to calm the wild fluctuations. The best thing to do, they said, would be to go back to my old friend NPH. This time we mixed it with regular insulin to quickly burn off the meals that caused my sugars to rise so rapidly. We also changed the time of my evening shot from nine o'clock to five thirty, which didn't bother me in the least. My diet was carefully controlled by the hospital staff, and they set up all the dosages. It was enjoyable to hand my control over to them, knowing that if any major mistakes were made they would be the Clinic's instead of mine. Throughout it all, I kept assuming that by the end of my stay I'd emerge a much healthier diabetic.

Although I did feel better on the new insulins, my charts didn't even out. Day after day they kept going haywire despite the best-controlled conditions in the world. I'd originally planned on staying for about five days, but ended up staying longer as we tried to master my diabetes.

"Well," the doctor in charge of my case finally said, "I don't think we can expect more than we've got. Your diabetes is fragile by nature, and it doesn't look as though we can really change that."

I trusted her more than I had many physicians in my past. All week long she had thrown her best into it, had worked with me every step of the way, and most of all, I could tell she wasn't trying to protect herself. I appreciated her careful work and felt she was an outstanding doctor. At first, her words were something of a relief. If the swings couldn't be prevented at the Joslin Clinic, then there were no logical reasons for me to hold myself accountable to a kind of fairy-tale diabetes in which everything went according to Hoyle. That recognition could have changed the whole name of the game.

Nevertheless, I hoped the new diet, insulin, and routines of the Clinic could be taken home and preserved. When Connie picked me up, I told her all about the complications I'd seen for the first time and stressed the need for better control. As we drove home we made plans to stop eating our meals at the school cafeteria, to take the food scale out of the closet and make a new start.

Within several months, our attempts had fallen by the wayside. I was back in the thick of things at school, and felt as if I would be "giving in" to myself if I spent too much time trying to maintain an even balance. Although I physically felt better than I had before going to Joslin, the middle ground between perfection and resenting the whole thing seemed impossible to find. The strange thing was that my power to "do something" about diabetes kept increasing. Just as magical thinking kept raising the stakes despite its obvious failures, my attempts at willpower did the same thing. I kept wanting to prove myself in an impossible battle and resented having to do so.

"Part of the reason that happened," said Dick, "was that you interpreted Joslin as being an ideal place. It wasn't ideal, but you thought it would be. So your perceptions kept feeding you information that you were denying. That created a bind that many diabetics face."

"What's the bind?" I asked.

"It came out like this. If the Clinic was ideal, and something was still wrong after they've been working on you, then you were the problem. Even after they told you that you weren't the problem, the equation still held true."

"So the anger would turn on myself?"

"Right," said Dick. "You were the bad guy, and to prove it, your diabetes screwed up. It has to fit."

It did.

30 ✦ BILL

Bill was a candidate for admission to the Hyde School. He came for his interview one March afternoon, and I was designated to sit in on the session. During the interview we tried to get to know each student as well as possible by exploring who he was, what he'd done, and the kind of person he wanted to become. As a sophomore, Bill hadn't done well in school. His performance ran a distant second to his expectations, and he seemed unable to get out of the rut. Nevertheless, we believed enough in what he wanted to do with life to offer him a spot.

"Do you think you really want to come here?" we asked near the end of the interview.

"Yes," said Bill, realizing that turning hopes into reality wouldn't be easy.

"Great," we said. "Is there anything else you want to bring up?"

"No," he said. There was a pause, and his mother, who had been with us throughout the interview, looked at her son sitting on the other side of the small office.

"Bill," she said, trying to remind him of something, "there's a skeleton you haven't mentioned."

"What?" said Bill. I suspect he would have disappeared on the spot if he could have. She raised her eyebrows, but he still didn't say anything.

"Your diabetes?" she said.

164

"Oh, yes," said Bill, "I'm diabetic." My heart nearly dropped to the floor. I knew very well why he hadn't brought it up, and realized that if he came to the Hyde School his diabetes would become an important issue for both of us.

"Mr. Pray is diabetic as well," said the interviewer almost immediately, "and he can really help you." His revelation brought forth no anger or embarrassment on my part, but it did make me wonder how on earth I'd help Bill.

"How are you doing with it?" I asked, knowing the answer already.

"Okay," said Bill without much enthusiasm.

"We'll have to talk more about it," I said. "All I can say to you is that you need to control it instead of letting it control you. That, as you probably know, is a lot easier said than done. But you're here to prepare for your future. If you want genuine confidence, you can't let as important a part of your life as diabetes be a hidden problem while working on 'the rest' of your life. The two need to go hand in hand."

Neither of us quite knew how to make those impressive words come true, but that afternoon we both accepted the goal. I told him the kitchen would make any necessary provisions, and that it would be all right for him to keep his equipment in his room. Looking for some kind of guideposts, I even mentioned that he should keep an accurate record book. Whenever I saw Bill over the next few years, diabetes would be the first thought that flashed through my mind. The same was true for Bill. Curiously enough, we kept our talks to how we were doing instead of what diabetes meant to us. Diabetes was a liability that needed to be conquered, and our desire for a solution didn't allow much room to share our real stories.

"The message I got from the interview," said Bill when I talked to him years after his graduation, "was that you guys were going to fix me. I had always assumed that if diabetes could be solved, the rest of my life would fall into place. But it was like I was a computer and you didn't know the right language."

"That's the same approach I took toward Joslin," I said. "So what was the right language?"

"In very many respects," said Bill, "I considered myself normal. But down deep I either didn't want to be diabetic at all or felt I needed to be that 'picture-perfect' diabetic which didn't exist. So both were impossible. The result was that being diabetic became an excuse to avoid any problem I chose to avoid.

"I always thought there was an unsaid reason for my being diabetic. In a journal I wrote a few years ago, I put it this way: 'When I was ten, I developed diabetes. Suddenly my world changed. Everything changed. But when I look at it now, it was my self-concept that changed. I was suddenly different from everybody else. I felt like I must have done something wrong, and this was my punishment. Only I didn't know what I had done. I was very confused.'

"As a result, I kept putting off coming to terms with diabetes. I can remember the regular promises I'd make to myself on my birthdays. I didn't share them with anyone, but would say to myself, 'Well, if by the time I am twenty-one I haven't become the perfect diabetic, then I'll need to question what I'm doing with my life.' Now I'm twenty-five, and it's like that starting line is still out there somewhere."

Diabetes had riddled Bill's family. Both his father and a sister were diabetic. They had been to the Joslin Clinic several times, and out of necessity knew the conventional wisdom of the disease. I had the feeling his mother had seen enough diabetes to last several lifetimes. I assumed that the presence of diabetes in his family would help in Bill's eventual acceptance. As it turned out, quite the opposite was true.

"A lot of the time," Bill said as he continued his story, "it felt like diabetes stifled deep communication in our family. Most of the time, there was a way around the tough questions. And our not dealing with it was part of my protection. My father wasn't the perfect diabetic either. He has gone for thirty years and still hasn't put it all together, so I thought, 'Why should I expect I'll be able to do it?' "

More than they realize, parents often hold the keys to what will and will not be explored in the lives of their children. As the expression goes, "The apple doesn't fall far from the tree." I thought back to a family conference I'd called before Bill's graduation. His year hadn't been bad, but neither had it been inspiring. We all sat down in an empty classroom to try to pull out the stops.

"It's time," I said, "for you to share as a family what this disease means to you. Every instinct I have tells me it's a sleeping giant. It is

166

for me too, and even though I've thought a lot about diabetes and my life, I don't know how to open things up because I haven't done it fully for myself. I do know that diabetes is central to Bill's life. I think it has kept him from taking confidence in himself, and I think he needs your help getting beyond the images of diabetes and trying to figure out where it fits in his life."

They all agreed. But, as in the story of the mice who all decided it would be a great idea to place a bell around the neck of the cat, who would bell the cat? And just what was the bell? I looked for a starting place, but my stories seemed weak. All I could do was come up with a diagnosis of the "problem." We knew diabetes was unexplored territory and had no idea how to proceed.

One rule in teaching is that you can't give what you don't have. If you're not willing to ask of yourself what is asked of others, teaching isn't much more than words. Teaching Bill challenged everything I had and made me more aware than ever that there was something about diabetes I didn't understand. It was an impasse that, just as Dick Evans had said, made me turn on myself in battles of willpower.

Bath is built along the western bank of the Kennebec River in coastal Maine. It is a historic New England town, filled with white houses and lovely streets. Each morning I'd go for a run down along the river. As I approached the Bath Iron Works shipyard, a predictable litany would match the pace of my run.

"Today is the day for a new beginning," the practiced thought always began. "Today is the day you'll get this thing licked. You know you can do it if you try. There will be no excesses, no excuses. You can move through the meals and take just what you need. The frustrating days are behind you. Follow the rules and the battle is won."

The lines came to me like creatures of habit. I'd usually keep the promises throughout the morning until an approaching reaction or an unscheduled event required a change in plans. Suddenly, I'd find myself playing catch-up ball. The urine test I'd planned on taking before lunch fell by the wayside. If the lunch looked good, as it usually did, I'd take an extra helping, figuring I'd burn it off that afternoon. In short, desire and a healthy appetite replaced the morning's ideal.

By late afternoon there would come a certain moment when I

could physically feel my resolve crumble entirely. Once it began to go, there was no calling it back. In fact, the gut rebellion had a certain pleasure connected with it. At dinner I'd eat with an abandon that would throw me off despite the few extra units of regular insulin I'd taken to allow for a larger meal. The exercise I had with my sports teams was a great excuse for almost any indulgence at dinner. When ten thirty rolled around, particularly if I'd been under a great deal of stress, a binge mentality frequently took over. Sandwiches, cookies, whatever we had in the icebox would be just fine. I would eat those foods to the tune of a two-sided nighttime litany.

"You're going to pay for this," said one side.

"What's the difference?" said the other. "You've earned it. And besides, you're already off kilter."

"Why are you doing this?" asked the first.

"Why not?" answered the second. "Tomorrow is another day, and it will be the new beginning." The next morning, in the beautiful city of Bath, the process began again.

Dick Evans began to laugh as I told him about the great debate.

"Do you know what this reminds me of?" he asked. "When I tried to quit smoking, I'd say to myself, 'This is definitely going to be my last cigarette.' Then an hour later I promised myself that the next cigarette would be the last one for sure. Mark Twain was right when he said quitting smoking was the easiest thing in the world because he had done it a thousand times.

"When you try to make a show of willpower, publicly or privately, it doesn't work. I am convinced human beings don't have that willpower."

"Why not?" I asked.

"Because that kind of willpower is based on proving something instead of accepting reality. It implies a spectacular end that happens more in the movies than in real life. It is like a champion boxer who has retired undefeated. After a while, he begins to question his identity, and wonders if he is still a champion. So he has to go out and fight, and will probably get the daylights beat out of him. But if he wins and retires again, just watch. It won't be long before he'll go out and try it again."

"Sounds like Ali," I said. "With me there really was an adversary relationship in there. It was like I was fighting myself."

168

"The willpower stage," said Dick, "is exactly that. It is a dialogue with one self, and it's a dialogue about Catch-22 impossibles."

"When those litanies ran through my mind," I said, "I knew they wouldn't work and suspected they would someday pass away. But they still carried a lot of power, and I couldn't get rid of them. Why not?"

"It's more heroic to fight than to be a picture-perfect diabetic," answered Dick. "Who wants to give in to something like diabetes? You'd really be a hero to yourself if you could in fact conquer it. But without the fight you lose your status as a hero. It's like television. Have you ever seen a show about preventive medicine that did well in the ratings? How did Bill see you?"

"He looked up to me as the ideal diabetic. He told me that he figured my blood sugars were virtually indistinguishable from those of everyone else. He saw me at work, and couldn't see what a struggle it all was."

"He saw you as the hero you hoped you could be. No wonder it was difficult for you to share your experiences with him. It's hard for someone who is drinking to tell someone else to stop drinking."

The conflict became clear. Whereas magical thinking was a battle of limits, willpower was a battle of expectations. My promises to myself involved a fantastic picture of the way diabetes should be. But genuine acceptance has little to do with outer appearances. It is an internal, deeply personal reconciliation of life, disease, and one's future. As long as I tried to be the hero on the basis of overcoming problems I had to accept, it wouldn't, couldn't, and didn't work.

The willpower stage occurs and recurs in the lives of most diabetics. I thought of a college kid who followed his diet but binged on beer, an older man who kept teasing the dietitian about the martini(s) he enjoyed in "moderation," and a gentleman who admitted to his complete acceptance of diabetes only to have his wife remind him of his twenty-year weight problem and his fondness for bowls of buttered popcorn. We all had our bouts with willpower, most of which we kept to ourselves.

"Your experience," said Dick, "is probably typical of many diabetics. The only part of it that is atypical is the degree of awareness that you had while you were going through it all. You had a tremendous awareness of your own processes. It's almost like you've studied yourself as an animal, and learned to accept the things you have to accept by studying yourself in an objective way. Your wanting to teach Bill raised the stakes a notch. Your instincts were right, even though you didn't know what to do with them.

"Many people try to live on the surface so they don't have to deal with those unresolved 'monsters' down deep within us. But my experience as a psychiatrist is that there aren't very many people who don't need to come to grips with themselves sometime during their life, be it early or late.

"I think diabetics have difficulty putting their struggles into perspective. When I was a kid I remember thinking it was almost unbearable to be named Richard. It isn't quite the same as being diabetic, but I wasn't sure if I was going to be able to survive that. From an adult's perspective, that sounds like a lot of foolishness.

"Take any individual from among the vast majority and follow them around for a couple of days, and you'll find they've got something comparable to diabetes as a problem to live with. Something about their identity will be engaged in a long, drawn-out hassle to learn the rules that work for them."

After Dick left, I thought about the evening Bill and I talked about diabetes and our lives, filling in the holes that had been missing for both of us when he was a student.

"You know," Bill had said as we finished our talk, "I guess in a sense I'm taking better care of myself than I usually give myself credit for. I usually don't feel that way. I've always approached it from the viewpoint of what I haven't done."

"That's the way it was for me, Bill," I said. "That's the way it was for me too."

170

31 ✦ HOMEWORK

We had been married six years before deciding to have kids. Part of our waiting was due to no more than the ordinary scruples of a marriage that wanted to make sure it would get off the ground. The rest of our hesitation was due to the laws of heredity. Because Connie didn't have diabetes anywhere in her family tree, our children would run about a 25 percent chance of becoming diabetic, though the certainty was 100 percent that they would inherit the trait. Although falling in love had erased any worries about getting married, having children seemed like a different matter entirely. Oddly enough, passing on the trait concerned me more than whether or not our children became diabetic themselves. Not knowing quite what to do about such a dilemma, we simply decided to wait.

One day, as I was in the midst of working with a group of parents, it suddenly occurred to me that the contributions one makes with one's life are more important than the health of the contributor. It was one of those simple observations that sometimes take a long time to see. Health isn't an end in and of itself, despite fads to the contrary. It merely provides the base upon which we express our lives.

With that in mind, we next learned that there was no sure way to find out whether or not Connie was a carrier despite her family tree, and that the Mendelian laws of genetics that could successfully predict the color of fruit fly wings didn't always work when it came to diabetes. Actually, I was glad to know the demanding laws didn't always work. We put our hesitation behind us, and one bright summer afternoon decided that the whole adventure was worth the risk.

When Connie became pregnant the following spring, we were so excited we scarcely knew what to do. We read fifty books on child-bearing, learned that few babies are ever born diabetic, sorted through thousands of potential names, wondered if "it" would be a boy or a girl, rearranged the house, and waited for slow time to pass quickly by. I finally understood why my friend Dave of "Dave's Diary" had spent so much time writing about his child-to-be.

Had Connie been the diabetic in our family, the wait might have been an entirely different matter. Diabetes could seriously jeopardize pregnancy. When a diabetic mother falls into a reaction or slips into a coma, so does the baby that is tied so closely to her system. The consequences could be deadly. The chance of miscarriage was so great that years ago many diabetic women were advised not to attempt to have children at all.

I'd heard of a girl who married in her late teens and whose diabetes wasn't in the best of shape. Just after her marriage, she decided to have herself sterilized. Although I knew none of the particulars, I couldn't help wondering if she had made her decision before she came to terms with her disease or before she had heard of the break-throughs that might have given her the chance for a safe pregnancy. The closer we came to the birth of our first, the more thankful I was that I hadn't let the intense self-doubts of an earlier age mark our future as a family.

Fortunately, some tremendous advances have been made in this area. Insulin pumps, for example, can now monitor blood sugars automatically and release insulin as needed through a needle that remains inserted beneath the skin. The ones I've seen are about the size of a walkie-talkie, and are attached to one's belt or pants. While they may be inconvenient, and while they may not be practical for every-day use, they are a godsend for pregnant diabetics. Some women are able to turn over a whole new leaf of self-control once they become pregnant. They know they're fighting for the life of their baby, and follow their regimens to the letter. Sometimes their control can be sustained after delivery; sometimes it can't.

Timothy Allan Pray, the first of our four kids, was finally born on a cold January night. When we went home a week later, we were as proud a pair of parents as there ever have been. Tim, just as the doctor had predicted, was not born diabetic. We, however, couldn't help keeping an eagle eye out for just how thirsty this little one might be. One day our sitter, who had been given explicit instructions about the warning signs of diabetes, gave us a call at school.

"Tim has been wetting his diapers a lot," she said.

"Here we go," I thought, imagining sopping diapers and constant streams of pale urine. I quickly found Connie and we ran home as though the house was on fire. She dug out the testing equipment from the back of a tool drawer and told me to wring out five drops from Tim's wet diaper. We gathered around the test and breathed a sigh of relief as the test turned out blue as blue could be.

Throughout Tim's first year, I couldn't help wondering how I'd someday tell him about diabetes. I figured he'd probably just grow up and one day notice I took shots that nobody else in the family seemed to need. He'd tell his friends about it, and they'd all be surprised, saying their dads didn't get to take shots. Or maybe he would ask why I didn't eat ice cream when we went to McDonald's. When he became old enough to understand, I didn't want to give him lectures or hide behind a phony model. Kids reflect the character of their parents as they grow. If I wanted him eventually to live his whole life with confidence, I simply had to do the same with mine, and diabetes was no exception.

In my professional life, everything was moving right along. I'd been director of the summer school, had created a number of new community programs, and was ready to launch into a new project involving parents. Part of the parents' curriculum involved their writing vignettes about their lives that could be shared with their kids. For some, alcohol was a prime concern.

It didn't take long to notice a sharp difference between those who had accepted their excessive drinking as a problem and those who hadn't. Those who didn't think they had a drinking problem usually had the best rationalizations in the world. Intellectually speaking, they knew all about the dangers of drinking too much. The more convinced they were, the less they heeded the concerns of their kids or spouse, and the more I noticed they were at war with themselves.

On the other hand, those who had accepted their alcoholism and went to Alcoholics Anonymous meetings had an altogether different countenance. They seemed to understand life on a deeper level. They could share stories that would have embarrassed the daylights out of them years earlier in a new and inspirational way. One man joked at a meeting that before AA his social drinking used to include sneaking into his garage at two thirty in the morning to find some booze. As he read his story and the other parents laughed (or held their breath), I thought about my excessive bedtime snacks that supposedly protected me from reactions in the middle of the night. I would have felt ashamed to tell anybody about those excesses. In fact, I'd even make sure Connie was asleep before heading for the kitchen. These people understood something about themselves, acceptance, and the nature of their disease.

From them I got an idea. Alcoholics who denied their alcoholism didn't get help. Diabetics who fought their disease weren't much different. We both were sick, especially when we tried to deny our diseases. But a deeper acceptance was possible. If I surrounded myself with people who had come to an acceptance of their disease, perhaps there was something I could learn.

Knowing my ability to rationalize, I decided to use diabetes, when I talked to the parents on the opening day of summer school, as an example of the kind of personal issue that families must face. Once I had told them, there was no way I could back out of my plan when the Friday-night AA meeting rolled around.

I felt like an intruder as I quietly walked into my first meeting. The room was filled with people sitting in the tan metal chairs that all churches seem to have, and almost everybody smoked and drank coffee as if it were going out of style. As people noticed me and said hello, I felt that they had the wisdom to look right through me and the common sense to know they shouldn't. When the meeting began, speakers stood up one after another and shared their stories. They had come to realize that drinking controlled them instead of the other way around. They talked about the unpredictable moment when they had suddenly realized they sincerely didn't want it that way. They talked about an acceptance that was deeper than logic. For them, it was a deeply personal and even spiritual matter. Their

174

stories made sense. Their lack of pretense was powerful. By the end of the evening, I knew that they and I shared a challenge, and that there was hope.

As the weeks went by, however, my feeling out of place continued. I told one veteran about my diabetes, and he acknowledged the link but couldn't say anything more. Alcoholics Anonymous was for alcoholics. It wouldn't have been right for me to stand up and share a story about diabetes.

Each week chips were given to alcoholics who were beginning the program and to those who had gone for a week, thirty days, or a year without drinking. Carried in the pocket like change, the chip was a steady reminder of their disease and that they needed help. For me, as a diabetic, there was no one chip I could carry. I would need, I joked to myself, a diet chip, an exercise chip, an insulin chip, a test chip, and even a record-book chip all at the same time! So while the meetings helped me recognize the elusive nature of acceptance, attending began to feel like a burden. One night, to my absolute delight, I was unable to find a parking space.

"Well," I said out loud, "it looks like you'll just have to go back home." By the time I came to the end of the driveway, my conscience caught up with me.

"You can't let yourself get away with this," I said to myself. I spun the car around, finally found a distant spot, and walked into the meeting with great resignation.

"You really put yourself through the paces, didn't you?" said Dick Evans after he heard my story.

"You're telling me!" I said with a smile. "That was a tough summer. But as I see it now, going to all those meetings was like doing homework. It was me against myself, but I think those cataclysmic battles were somehow necessary."

"They should be expected," Dick said emphatically. "Those wrestlings and rebellions were essential. You had to convert old approaches into new ways of seeing yourself as a person and as a diabetic. It was similar to the process alcoholics go through when they're ready to stop drinking."

"There are no twelve easy steps to diabetic acceptance and control," I said. "So one message we can give is that doctors and patients shouldn't be overly threatened if they have a tough time working it all out."

From a logical viewpoint, the battles of willpower seem just as foolish as the battles of magical thinking. After all, all an alcoholic has to do to stop drinking is stop drinking. All a diabetic has to do is conform to the rules and regulations of diabetes. But life, thank heaven, isn't that simple. Coming to terms with oneself isn't a matter of conformity. It is a matter of discovering a sense of one's uniqueness, one's character, and one's commitment as a man or a woman. Just as there are no surefire easy answers in life, there are no quick answers for acceptance.

"AA doesn't allow much for the heroics of willpower," said Dick. "In fact, the first of their twelve steps recognizes their powerlessness over alcohol."

"That is precisely how I felt about my diabetes," I said, "but I couldn't give in. I kept thinking I had to do something first."

"That's the problem," said Dick. "You were always focusing on what you hadn't done, and denied yourself in the process."

"I had to accept myself," I said to Dick.

"As less than perfect," he said, finishing the thought. "And that happens to be an essential lesson for all of us whether or not we're diabetic."

"At the end of that summer school," I said, "the kids told me during evaluations that while they deeply respected and trusted me, they didn't quite know who I was. They couldn't quite identify with me as a person."

"That had a lot to do with your diabetes," said Dick. "You had a tendency to try and be so 'right' so much of the time. Diabetes is something you couldn't do anything about. To compensate for that, you tried to be more than perfect in every other way—much more so than most other young adults feel they ever have to be.

"Trusting yourself was difficult because you might be rejected, you might be judged because you weren't perfect. And now that you were a father, your wanting to pass something solid on to Tim added fuel to the fire."

"How so?" I asked.

"You've said before that you felt you didn't have much time in life.

176

But I think what you meant and didn't say is that you have to cover more ground than an ordinary person in order to make up for the diabetes. AA helped you realize you needed to set your own pace. You were a successful teacher and the director of summer school, but the real battle was for your own identity. That's an inevitable stage of human growth."

"Pretty heavy stuff," I said.

"It's like navigating along the Maine coast in a fog," said Dick with a laugh. "You go from sounder to sounder."

I had always told kids during their interviews that if a person keeps on doing things he already knows he can do, he may be getting older rather than growing up. It was advice that had served me well, and now it needed to be applied again. I had to grow beyond what I knew to discover the full range of my character and creativity.

"Connie," I said one night, "I'm going back to Joslin. I don't know exactly how, but it's time to put this thing away once and for all."

We called the Clinic, found it had an opening the day after Christmas, 1978, and signed up. The wrestling was over, my due bills paid. Now it was time to find out.

32 ◆ RELEASE

"Doctor," I said to the energetic intern who gave me my initial physical at Joslin, "let me tell you why I'm here. I think there is a relationship between alcoholism and diabetes, and I'm like the alcoholic who hasn't stopped drinking. I'm sick and tired of the battles and have come to end them."

"Good luck," he said as though the quest for the Holy Grail wasn't a particularly productive search. My words felt forced, but nobody could help if he didn't know why I was there, so I pulled out all the stops.

"I began going to some AA meetings last summer," I said, "and for a while they helped."

"Good," he said briskly. "It sounds like you're pretty intense about it." Intensity was one quality I had more of than I knew what to do with. I suppose I expected him to give me some counseling, to tell me to check into another hospital, or to stop in his tracks in acknowledgment of my stupendous remark. He, of course, merely finished my exam and went on his way. It bothered me that he didn't seem to understand, but then he was only a young intern.

When my doctor came in, I brought up the subject again. Halfway through my speech, the same thing happened. The more I spoke, the more I felt the profound separation that had begun with the trip to Maine so many years before.

"What you're talking about," he finally said, "we call acceptance.

You have to accept your disease." Then he continued the exam much as the intern had before him, as though stating the problem could resolve it. It hit me like a ton of bricks that although he was correct in his diagnosis, he hadn't perceived the dilemma. It's not that he wasn't interested, because he was. And it's not that I wasn't coherent, because my words did make logical sense. I already knew I had to come to terms with diabetes. But just how does one do that?

I had the feeling my search was supposed to be kept private. It was as though the entire system of treatment avoided the acceptance process that is so integral to the life of a diabetic. Medical advice alone wasn't enough to reconcile an individual's life and the constraints of disease. And yet most books and guides and the Clinic itself focused on the mechanics of treatment while neglecting the inevitable and intangible battles of acceptance. For me it was a breathtaking realization. I'd thought there might be an answer somewhere, and there wasn't. If there was to be a breakthrough, I'd have to find it on my own.

Talking with other diabetics at the Clinic seemed the best way to begin. We were quite an assortment. A lawyer from New York, a teacher from New Jersey, a Long Island businessman, a young girl from Indiana about to be married, and a man who wanted to make nightly excursions into Boston's red-light Combat Zone made up the cast of characters. Our battles with willpower, our speculation about possible cures, the stories of our reactions, and our fear of potential complications all brought us together. We liked the ideal arrangements at the Clinic, yet realized how different it was from our lives in the "real" world.

One day two interns stopped by with clipboards in hand and asked me to describe how I felt when my sugars ran high. I was glad they'd asked, because most of the time I was supposed to be learning from them and I enjoyed the chance to give something back.

"Well," I said, trying to find words to express the feelings exactly, "my blood thickens. It gets heavy, as though it turns into a puffy syrup. Then I get tired, sleepy, and claustrophobic. But mostly it's that thick feeling in my blood."

"See," said the intern as though he'd just hit the jackpot, "that's how they all describe it." If looks could kill, I'd have had him six feet

179

under. Who was he to describe "us" as a group? Who was he to ask for a sincere answer and then glibly toss it into his list of probable answers? He made me so angry I could hardly see straight for a moment. After they left, however, I realized that his manners weren't the real problem. In what was to be my last fling with the anger of denial, I simply didn't want to be tagged diabetic.

After a few days, there came to Joslin a woman who had a different kind of air about her. She was from Connecticut and set up shop in the Clinic with the firm resolve of an old pro. Even though she was there to receive a hookup for kidney dialysis, she didn't seem afraid. As I remember it, she knitted and had brought her work with her. One day as she was sitting in the lounge, I went over to talk with her.

"How long have you been diabetic?" I casually asked. That was always the best opening question, and usually gave me the upper hand.

"Fifty years," she said. I could scarcely believe my ears.

"Fifty years?" I said. "There aren't many of you around!" She smiled at my astonishment and told me she had been an early patient of the famed Dr. Joslin himself. She joked that her half-century's worth of charts made a file twice the size of the New York City telephone directory.

"I'm one of their favorites," she said with a smile. She had been diabetic nearly twice as long as I'd lived, and I wanted to glean all she had learned.

Her story wasn't very long, and it wasn't even particularly poignant. She had developed diabetes at an early age and had seen breakthroughs come and go. She had married and had several children. From the way she spoke, she was neither overly concerned about her diabetes nor trying to avoid it. I admired her ease and honesty.

"Listen," I said with an urgent tone to my voice, "let me tell you what bothers me about diabetes." I told her about the promises made and promises broken, that diabetes ruled me more than I ruled it, that I wanted to teach Tim to be honest with his life when I couldn't be entirely honest about mine. I told her about my job, how much I loved teaching, and the changes in education we hoped to make.

"Starting next month," I said, "I'm going to be traveling a lot. I want to go, but have got to get things in order." It had all spilled out, and then there wasn't much more to say. At that point she stopped her knitting and looked up.

"Do you know what I would do if I were you?" she asked.

"What?" I said. At that moment, a funny thing happened. I had absolutely no idea what she was going to say. In most conversations about diabetes I could accurately predict what I was going to hear. The advice of doctors and my own expectations ran through my mind like prerecorded messages of moral and medical advice. But when she asked me that question, I found myself unexpectedly listening.

"Forget it," she said; "just forget it. You are a young man with a family, with imagination, with lots you want to do. Do it, and don't worry about the diabetes." For some reason, I believed her. She'd expressed the one option I'd never considered. I'd always thought the solution to diabetes lay in "doing something." The solution, she seemed to say, lay in trusting my strength and vision as a person. She wasn't saying diabetes should be ignored, nor that it should be attacked as though it could be conquered. She was saying I needed to accept myself.

"Look," she said, "when you were eighteen did you ever cheat on your diet?"

"Sure," I said

"So did I. But that didn't last forever. I grew up. There is no reason diabetes should hold you back."

I am generally skeptical of people who say they have suddenly seen the light, but in a quiet sort of way that is what happened. On my journey, she was the helper who unexpectedly appeared and allowed the pieces to fall into place. It was a feeling of recognition. When my childhood friend *Paddle-to-the-Sea* became stuck in a log and headed toward the blades of a sawmill, a worker reached down and pulled him to safety just when all was about to be lost. When Jonah was thrown into the sea, there came a great fish. When Dorothy in *The Wizard of Oz* wanted to go back to Kansas, she learned she'd had the secret right with her all the time. And her friends the lion, the tin man, and the scarecrow already had within them the qualities they were searching for. Oz simply helped them accept the strengths they already had. So it was with me.

Her advice made for a paradox. Only by forgetting diabetes could I look in a mirror and see myself as a diabetic. As that happened, diabetes became a teacher instead of a threat, and the artificial separation between my life and my disease became reconciled.

On the last day of my stay, my doctor came in for his final visit. He looked content.

"Whatever you've been doing all these years," he said, "keep doing it. You're in great shape." He smiled, and my spirits soared. The fights and battles had paid off with a pleasing assurance.

When Connie came on December 31 to pick me up, it was difficult at first to describe to her what had happened. The results, however, soon became plain to both of us. The compulsive binges ended. Balancing diet, insulin, and exercise was no longer a burden. Diabetes, which had for so long been a matter of success or failure, simply became a gently accepted fact. The heroic battles trying to prove my willpower faded away as though they were no longer needed. I felt more mature, and took increased pride in who I was. Instead of separating me from others, diabetes helped me bridge the gap. I discovered that sharing my experience battling with intangibles could inspire others with their own growth. I learned again and again that my struggles with acceptance weren't much different from the struggles others face as they grow and come into their own. And most important of all, I could talk about my diabetes as though it actually belonged to me.

A year later when I returned to Joslin, I made sure to see the doctor I'd spoken with about acceptance. I saw our talk as a kind of test. If I choked on my words or explained without sharing, it might indicate I'd been talking to myself too much despite the improvement. If we could communicate, then I could further trust the depth of my story. Either way, I knew I couldn't fake it.

When I asked if we could talk for a moment at the end of my exam, he readily agreed. I spent perhaps ten minutes telling him what had happened, about how tricky acceptance could be and how central it was in a diabetic's life. After a while he smiled.

"You have one of those needling Yankee consciences, don't you?" he said. "Are you from Maine?"

"No," I said, "I was brought up in Colorado." We both laughed.

He had listened carefully, and the distance I had hoped wouldn't be there never came between us. He later corresponded with me as I tried to give back to the Clinic the insights I'd gained. He had spent his life caring for diabetics and knew how important acceptance could be. I had spent my life working toward acceptance and knew how important good care could be. We both recognized that one without the other could never do the job.

33 · TWO STORIES

I have intentionally not talked much about religion in these stories. Thoughts of being miraculously healed and released from the labyrinth of life and disease make me uncomfortable. There may be miracles through which diabetics have been cured, just as there are stories of families whose test of faith resulted in a lost child. Somewhere between the instant cures and lost lives, however, I suspect that most diabetics do turn to religion at one time or another for help.

I certainly did. For me, learning to accept diabetes taught me something about prayer. I had asked for an end to my rebellions, for the willpower to conquer diabetes, for deliverance from something instead of the courage to accept the truth. It reminds me of someone who, once dealt a hand of cards, works overtime to change the deck. When it can't be changed, he still fully expects four aces and a wild card in every hand of five-card stud. When they don't show up, anger carries the day. To then pray for aces doesn't make much sense. In hindsight, praying for strength to overcome diabetes doesn't make much sense either.

After the doctor told me to just keep on doing whatever I'd been doing, I wound my way through the tunnels of Joslin to the chapel at Deaconess Hospital. There was no one there, so I walked in with a full heart. The stained-glass windows were filled with bright colors as I sat there with a sense of relief and thanks. I felt that a whole phase of my life was at an end. The desire to overcome something was replaced with a recognition of a journey that had taught me so much about myself, my disease, and my faith. There would be new battles, but they wouldn't be me against diabetes. I felt stronger.

Walking back to the Clinic, I noticed a couple with a young boy slowly strolling down the hallway. They were clearly upset about something. The father had his arm around his son's shoulders. The boy, perhaps seven or eight years old, didn't look especially worried, but he was the object of their attention.

"Is something the matter?" I asked, approaching them. The father looked up.

"We've just found out that he's diabetic," he said. His wife had been fighting back the tears and suddenly began to cry again. The boy didn't say anything. In that moment I wanted to take all I had learned and share it with them.

"I'm diabetic too," I said with the exuberance I so deeply felt, "and I have been for twenty-two years." They looked at me as though it were impossible to have been diabetic for twenty-two years and still have spirit.

"It hasn't been easy," I said, "but I'm still here. I have a wife, a boy who's just about two, and I learned today that I don't have a trace of complications. It looks difficult, but the odds aren't insurmountable."

It turned out she was a nurse and had taken care of diabetic patients. Now that the patient was her son, all the training in the world didn't make much of a difference. Her husband was a contractor. His strength held things together as they tried to understand the risks and dangers of diabetes. Their eyes showed both affection for their son and concern for his future. There were so many things that could go wrong.

"I'm so scared," she said, fighting back the tears again. Her fears were clearly real. They were the same fears my mother had faced when she learned of my diabetes for the first time. The look in the boy's eyes took me back to that summer in Maine when it seemed my life really began. It was as though one journey had ended and another had just begun.

I tried to set them at ease, to tell them about diabetes support groups in their area, and that the challenge was to grow with diabetes and to learn from it. Fear, I told them, could only make matters worse. But not much sank in. In many ways, it couldn't have. A more powerful learning had already begun. Diabetes was a disease, and diseases were bad. Diabetes needed to be fought, and statistics proved the point. The parents had learned that diabetes is the third-leading cause of death, and that juvenile diabetes is the most serious type. The messages had set up the confrontation it had taken me so long to reconcile. Diabetes, a disease that must eventually be accepted and lived with, had already become for them a feared enemy.

Two years after seeing that family, I was talking with the director of the New England affiliate of the American Diabetes Association about my hopes for this book and the contradictions inherent in diabetes treatment. The organization had just come out with a new poster. It showed an attractive girl giving herself a shot in the arm. The caption read, "Every day of her life, Lisa Hendrickson fights a killer."

"What do you think of it?" asked the director.

"The poster," I said after a moment, "is the problem. It may be a great fund raiser, but it isn't for diabetics."

"If your children were diabetic, would you want them to see it?" she asked.

"No," I said, "but not for the reasons you suspect. If my kids become diabetic, I would want them to understand the complications and mechanics of their disease, much as I have come to understand them for myself. They would need to know the facts. But instead of seeing diabetes as an enemy, I would want them to learn to accept it, to grow with it, to see it as a teacher more than a handicap. Instead of separating themselves from their disease, I'd want them to learn not to make a distinction.

"That's what I had to learn, and it was the greatest lesson of my life."

That's what I had tried to say to the family who had just learned about their son's diabetes. And that's why my prayers were those of thanksgiving.

34 · CONCLUSION

This has been a story of acceptance. But it is also a story of growing up. After my return from Joslin, I began to feel more mature. For me, diabetes precipitated the journey, focused the issues that had to be faced, and eventually gave back as much as it took, or more. If I hadn't been diabetic, the challenges of growing up would still have been there, but they would have taken a different form. That's the joy of learning. We are all different, and yet we face universal challenges.

It is remarkable to me how rarely we share these adventures. I've always thought there was more to life than met the eye, and yet so much of our learning is centered around the tangible. In diabetes, for example, we are taught specific methods, as though acceptance comes as an automatic fact. In education as a whole, we often use tests to compare us with somebody else's standards of excellence. We hope that the truth will be positive, fear it will be negative, and sometimes don't find out what the truth actually "is." Intentionally or unintentionally, the setting of objective standards can conflict with the unique journey that all of us face as we grow and mature, whatever our age.

If you are diabetic, hopefully you'll identify with this story not because it is just like yours, but because between the lines of what "should be" you have your own story. The next chapter is expressly for you. If you're not diabetic, it doesn't really matter. Are these challenges different from someone's setting up his own business for the first time? From the love and drama of raising children? From losing a parent, a job, or any other action or consequence that requires faith?

I originally thought a book about acceptance would help diabetics, epileptics, and any individual or family that has to come face to face with a disease. I also hoped it would point out what I consider to be a glaring educational error in the conventional approaches. Acceptance is more than half the battle. But Dick and I soon realized we were really writing a book about education. How we all face the intangible questions that so deeply move, inspire, and sometimes depress us as people forms our character. Education is more than a matter of conformity. It is a matter of coming to terms with our potentials, responsibilities, and commitments.

So what should be changed? The point isn't to entirely undo the tests, competitions, and systems we already have. I am deeply thankful for the good work of the Joslin Clinic, for the organizations that work with diabetics, and for the books and magazines that helped me out along the way. But we must recognize the importance of applying the "answers" within the context of individual lives. I had to "undo" a system of thought before I could take its best parts and apply them. As I did, I came to a deeper appreciation of both my uniqueness and my disease. Diabetes could then become a teacher that engaged my spirit and challenged my potential. This was the journey.

If I could do it all over again, I'd make my journey less private. I'd try to gather the honest stories of how other people actually grew up. And I'd try to better realize that while health is very important, giving back and sharing one's commitment is more important.

In the future, I hope we will see the dilemmas of diabetes, or disease, or life, as opportunities for growth. That we can increasingly share the pool of experience we all have. And that we will begin to center education upon the capacity for growth, discovery, and commitment within each of us.

What does that have to do with diabetes? A lot. What does it have to do with growing up? Everything.

Postscripts

35 ✦ *FOR THE DIABETIC*

Given the unique nature of people, your journey through diabetes is different from mine. It is filled with the humor, the frustrations, the tough times, and the unexpected breakthroughs that have made your life what it is. Some of the lessons it took me a long time to learn you may have understood a long time ago. And what was a given for me may be difficult for you.

But that's not to say there aren't stages we share, and common lessons we'll come to understand in our own way. Denial, magical thinking, and willpower will probably show up in your life at one time or another. Accepting diabetes, whether you follow a "free" approach or test your blood three times a day and weigh out every serving, is a deeply personal matter. It is easier said than done. The ready-made answers didn't work for me, and I suspect they may not work for you either. Acceptance takes a lot of work, a lot of trials, a lot of realizing what we can and cannot change. For me, the lessons were quite the opposite of what I expected.

"What have you learned from being diabetic?" I once asked a diabetic.

"I've learned something about taking charge and running my life, or not taking charge and being tossed around. Most of all, I've learned that I can do whatever I want to do. And that means anything."

"I would have said the same thing once," I said, "but as it turned

191

out, diabetes taught me quite the opposite. I learned I can't do everything."

"What do you mean?" he asked.

"It taught me I can't wish things away, that my expectations can cloud the truth. When I came to see that diabetes can be a valued partner, it helped me accept my vision as a person. At one stage of the game I tried to conquer it, and found I couldn't. That was the failure that forced me to grow up."

I would not ask you to see diabetes as a friend from the beginning. Appealing as the idea might seem, it isn't that simple. I remember the day I hoped the doctor would say no more insulin was necessary, the day I tried to wish it all away, and the day I saw some of the battles resolved. It took a long time. I do believe, however, that the extent to which you see diabetes as an enemy or a friend may well mark the extent to which you've accepted it.

Working with others can help. It took a long time before I realized my struggles were common to other diabetics. If you can find a group where diabetics honestly share their stories, attend some meetings and see what happens. You may be surprised how your experiences can inspire others and how much you can learn. Remember that an understanding of the techniques and mechanics is essential, but just as important is the way you see yourself and your personal growth.

Like a story that seems to change every time it is read, the challenges of diabetes keep popping up. I have recently been attending some meetings for diabetics at our city hospital. Every other week we gather to share our stories. There have been some tears, a good bit of laughter, and amazement at how much we're the same.

At our last meeting the hospital's nurse brought in a new portable blood-sugar monitoring kit. Several families had been using the kit with some success. Suddenly everyone in the room was wondering how much it cost and where it could be ordered. The more excited they became, the more reticent I began to feel. The machine cost a lot of money. I didn't have the time. I felt just fine without using it. I could feel myself digging in my heels at the thought of disbanding my internal radar system for the sake of technology, much the way Paul Bunyan scorned engines.

Walking out of the meeting, I knew why I'd been resistant.

Thoughts of my record books, unacceptable blood-sugar readings from the past, and the guilt that came with each poor reading all raced through me. For a moment, my desire to protect twenty-seven years' worth of learning overcame my wanting to find out what could happen with a new approach. Several days later, we put in an order for the machine.

If you don't quite know how you feel and aren't sure what to say when someone looks you squarely in the eye and says, "Tell me about your diabetes," don't worry about it. Most of us have been there at one time or another.

Once in the school we were writing "papers" about our lives. That sounded like a fairly simple task until we tried it, and found ourselves using our "perspectives and opinions" as a shield against our genuine feelings. I tried to write about my life by picking out those vivid moments which proved how unusual I really was. In the first draft, I didn't even mention diabetes. Needless to say, that paper didn't get off the ground. When in a second draft I included diabetes, it sounded like a collection of do's and don'ts blended with a healthy dose of denial.

Several days later, I sequestered myself in an office and began to write. I don't remember the line, but do remember my feelings welling up inside as I began to write the story of my diabetes. The feelings surprised and then reassured me. There was a well of experience to draw from.

To start, sit down with a piece of paper and begin to write your story. Leave out the mechanics, because you know them already. Start off by asking yourself what diabetes has taught you. Then write the incidents, the scenes, the hopes and fears with as much detail as you can find. See how honest you can be. See where your story takes you. If you want to share it, go ahead. If you don't, keep it for yourself. When you hit points of truth, it may seem that the paper almost writes itself.

There are few diabetics I've met who don't feel special in some way because of their diabetes. I know I do. My curiosity, my awareness, my desire to "do something," and the will to try to do it were all enhanced by diabetes. Growing up with a disease meant growing up in a way that made me feel special and unique. For that I'm thankful, despite all the tough times. Hopefully, the difference you feel as a diabetic will lead and guide you as a person.

I've always admired the Helen Kellers of the world. They have always seemed to give back more than they take. They aren't out to "prove themselves." Their conditions have helped form their character. Would Helen have wanted to see? I'm sure she would have. And yet the vision of a woman who couldn't see changed the way people saw. She wasn't a heroine because she vanquished her handicap and joined the ranks of "normal" people. She knew what she had, and knew the kind of person she wanted to be. Blindness or diabetes isn't inspiring in and of itself. But as we learn to grow and accept, our life with it can be.

Keep in mind that as a diabetic you're getting double messages all the time. You're supposed to accept a disease that's a killer, and lead a normal life while juggling twelve balls nobody else thinks about. You'll be expected to apply logic when the growth process is anything but logical. Reconciling such opposites is part of growing up regardless of your age. The conflict involves forms and reflects your character. Give it a chance, and diabetes may bring home some lessons others may learn much later in life.

Most of all, don't lose courage if you're having a tough time. Someday you may look back at yourself and wonder how on earth you could have been so far off base. If that happens, it's a good sign. You've grown and found the strength of character that was there all along. Get the best medical help you can, grow with diabetes, and when all seems lost just keep putting one foot in front of the other.

"Diabetes," I said to Dick as we wrapped up our work, "is a part of one's journey through life."

"Realizing that," said Dick, "seems to be the crux of the whole thing. As long as you were trying to force a square peg into a round hole, it wouldn't work. That's why diabetes helped you accept yourself as a person."

"That seems so simple," I said. "It was right there in front of me. I think it's there for every diabetic."

"Simple things," said Dick, "are hard to communicate and realize. Look how long it took you to see things from a different perspective. Communicating from one intellect to another is easy enough, but ac-

194

cepting and absorbing it is quite another challenge. Our message is that it is possible to come to terms with yourself as a diabetic, and to move from denial toward acceptance."

"So don't be afraid," I said, thinking of the family I'd met that afternoon at Joslin.

"Once you get there," said Dick, "it can be very rewarding. You're not going to fall through the bridge. It will hold."

"It has held," I said.

"And you can get across it."

36 ◆ FOR THE FAMILY

You have a story too. Denial, magical thinking, the desire to set things "right," and the confusions that come with each can affect your lives as much as the life of the diabetic in your family. Developing a genuine acceptance is a challenge for all of you.

Most families know the kind of people they'd like to be, and work to maintain that ideal. When something like diabetes comes along, the ideal is tested. The difference between "what we expected" and "what we got" comes sharply into focus.

"With diabetes," said Dick, "a whole new challenge came into your family. In spite of your being good and responsible people, it wouldn't go away no matter how hard you worked. That upset everyone. But because anger was seen as a fault, it was denied, went underground, and seeped out in other ways. For you, being 'positive' was easier than accepting it."

"When parents are filled with concern for their child," I said, thinking of my family, "it is tough to admit something like anger. It doesn't seem right to be angry at someone you love just because he's diabetic. Admitting that would seem like a failure."

"Well," Dick replied, "remember how you felt that admitting to diabetes would be an admission of defeat? It's like a farmer who feels the fox is bad because he steals a chicken. That's an absurd thought. Foxes steal chickens because that's the way foxes are built. But it is hard for humans, especially idealistic ones, to realize that feelings of anger are perfectly normal. That's the way people are built.

"It would have been helpful if your family could have understood their anger and realized that in spite of it they did a fine job as parents. They had to come to terms with diabetes much the way you did."

The challenge of acceptance can't be disguised behind our notions of "good" and "bad." "Good" families seem to take everything in stride. Their children grow up feeling "normal" and diabetes doesn't get in their way. "Bad" families feel sorry for themselves, ignore the rules, and see disease as a handicap. While the positive approach is probably the better of the two, both approaches are struggles with acceptance, and it is important to recognize the blind spots in each. Some "positive" families are afraid of feelings. To protect themselves, they turn their energies toward proving their strength at the expense of discovering how much there is to share. Other families become mired in guilt which prevents them from facing the facts.

It may be comforting to realize that the "perfect diabetic parent or spouse" who resides so actively in your imagination doesn't really exist. You can't help walking on pins and needles a bit during reaction-prone times. I doubt any parent can read about complications and not want to deny them. It isn't easy to figure out when a mood swing is due to an impending reaction and when it is nothing more than a stormy moment. The family that thinks it can handle everything without the slightest hitch is kidding itself.

So where do you start? See how much you can share. While you may think it is a sign of weakness, it may be reassuring to your son or daughter, husband, wife, or parent. Although I was in my twenties, I remember my sense of relief when my mother mentioned that she was beginning to realize the impact of diabetes on our family. After years of being strong, we were beginning to share.

If you don't know where to start, write a paper as described in Chapter 35. Or talk with the parents and spouses of other diabetics, whose experiences make for a great resource. Chances are you will learn a lot, and can develop a sense of humor which will stand you in good stead.

I suspect diabetes isn't something you just decide to talk about. It's my experience that most organized family sessions don't get off the ground unless there's a real emergency. I remember my father saying to me around my fourteenth birthday that the two of us should go rabbit hunting together. As soon as the words were out of his mouth I knew it was going to be a talk about sex, and my prediction was right on the money. I don't remember much of what we talked about, but do know we were equally nervous about the whole thing. If that kind of nervousness comes up when you approach the subject of diabetes, don't be surprised. Just forge ahead and keep in mind that there's a difference between growing up (whatever your age) and having a perfect approach. The double message that acceptance doesn't happen in a day and that touchy subjects shouldn't be avoided for too long a time binds you and the diabetic in your family together.

It may be difficult even to think about an eventual acceptance when there seem to be rebellions on all sides. What should you do when a teen-ager's diabetes is on the brink of disaster? How can you stand back and chalk one up for growing pains? There isn't an easy answer, but that's true for all parenting. How do you guide an adolescent without getting in the way? Be honest, recognize the struggles for what they are, take a good look at your own attitudes and expectations, and keep in mind that you're not alone.

Remember too that diabetes is a matter of juggling many variables. As a parent, you may assume a snack is needed every day at three o'clock when the diabetic in your family knows it isn't necessary at all. It's tough not to jump in and run everything according to rules and regulations, but what looks like a lax attitude to you may be no more than preventive medicine.

If your spouse is diabetic, remember the serenity prayer. Connie's learning not to "take care" of me strengthened our marriage. If your child is diabetic, keep in mind that the responsibility for good care must increasingly move from your shoulders to your child's. It is, after all, his or her life. If you end up with too much of the responsibility, or take too much of the credit, it won't work. The job of any parent is both to guide *and* to slowly let go. Diabetes must never be an excuse to avoid stepping out.

In our family, there were stages of letting go that were understood by all of us. Giving myself my own shots let me know from the beginning that the responsibility was mine. Joining Scouts, the first overnight in the mountains, leaving home, and going abroad were all mileposts. Each had an inherent risk, and each carried with it an added responsibility. For me, each was the beginning of a whole new adventure with diabetes and life.

There may eventually be a cure. I hope there is. But if I had sat back and waited for someone else's cure, it would have been a twenty-nine-year wait when there were better things to do. If you pour too much energy into waiting for a cure, you may end up denying the reality your son or daughter, husband or wife, brother of sister, lives with every day. It is tough enough to accept a disease that is billed as a dreaded killer. When the family hopes are based on a someday cure instead of one's developing one's potential, it can be more difficult still.

Finally, don't ever give up. The road to acceptance can be just as meaningful for you as it is for the diabetic in your family. While diabetes was a burden for our family in some ways, it also pulled us together. Looking back on it, I'm grateful for both.

37 ♦ *FOR THE DOCTOR*

I admire your patience. It must be frustrating and discouraging when your desire to help with the best medical training is short-circuited by a patient's battles with intangibles. Bill's analogy of diabetes' being like a computer for which nobody knows the proper language is often apt.

It is not the point of this book to prescribe a medical program for diabetic care. There are plenty of methods of care available. Clinics have developed programs; research and technology are finding new and effective ways to treat the wild fluctuations I battled with for so many years. Nevertheless, learning to accept diabetes as an integral part of one's growth is a challenge faced by every diabetic regardless of the approach used. In turning diabetes from an enemy into a teacher, you play an essential but difficult role.

"I think," said Dick, "that the medical community needs to understand that the wrestling process that seems so contrary to the best interests of a diabetic is essential to gaining a genuine understanding. In anatomical terms, a diabetic must eventually convert knowledge of the disease from the dominant to the nondominant hemisphere. So the problem isn't how do we eliminate that step, but how do we facilitate it."

The dominant hemisphere, as you already know, is the left side of the brain. Dick explained to me that it is in charge of functions such as memorized arithmetic and logical reasoning. The nondominant hemisphere is in charge of intuitive and conceptual processes. It lets us come up with answers to problems without having gone through the process of solving them. It allows for a musician to play a piece of music without thinking about each note, or for a skilled athlete to perform with consummate grace and skill without logical processes going on at all.

"That conversion," said Dick, "first means testing the limits of every aspect of the disease. It is important, without hurting yourself, to discover what those limits are. Then and only then can the rules and regulations of diabetes be applied as a natural part of one's life. In your case, Larry, you struggled with diabetes for a long time in a linear cognitive fashion without much apparent success while you checked out all the possible shortcuts and denials. Then you finally came to a nondominant-hemisphere acceptance."

I hesitate to give advice on how doctors should do their job, but I do hope this book has shown diabetes from a patient's point of view. For one reason or another, very few of these stories made it into my doctors' offices. To lay blame for that is a fruitless exercise. I believe we have all accepted an approach to treatment that doesn't take into account the growth process that is so essential in living with a disease like diabetes. Unless the acceptance process can somehow be recognized as part of the overall treatment, your knowledge as doctors may go unused until it is too late.

As Dick and I were trying to imagine how the doctor–patient relationship might be set up, I heard it like this:

"I've given you the mechanics," the doctor would say. "How you put them all together is going to be quite a challenge. You are going to learn more about yourself than many other people, which is good. You may wish you hadn't ever been diabetic in the first place, which is understandable. And you'll probably try to turn the clock back, which won't work no matter how hard you try.

"The only person who can put all this together on a daily basis is you. It may take a long time to fully realize that, but the journey begins now. Along the way, I hope you'll teach me what diabetes means to you."

"That is excellent," said Dick. "The only thing I would add is that it is essential not to try to be perfect. I don't mean that good control

201

isn't important, because it most certainly is. But perfection to a diabetic may not have a whole lot to do with the growth that enhances good care. Perfection is usually short-lived, and diabetes lasts a lifetime."

It isn't easy to balance your teaching and healing responsibilities, and you probably have to do it differently with each patient. However it is done, the doctor–patient relationship should result in mechanics and genuine acceptance going hand in hand.